Social Skills and Health

Other books by Michael Argyle

The Scientific Study of Social Behaviour (1957)
Religious Behaviour (1958)
Social Psychology through Experiment (with G. Humphrey) (1962)
Psychology and Social Problems (1964)
The Psychology of Interpersonal Behaviour (1967, 1972, 1978)
Social Interaction (1969)
The Social Psychology of Work (1972)
Social Encounters (1973)
Bodily Communication (1975)
The Social Psychology of Religion (with B. Beit-Hallahmi) (1975)
Gaze and Mutual Gaze (with M. Cook) (1976)
Social Skills and Mental Health (with P. Trower and B. Bryant) (1978)
Person to Person (with P. Trower) (1979)
Social Situations (with A. Furnham and J. A. Graham) (1981)

Social Skills and Health

EDITED BY
MICHAEL ARGYLE

METHUEN
London and New York

First published in 1981 by
Methuen & Co. Ltd
11 New Fetter Lane, London EC4P 4EE

Published in the USA by
Methuen & Co.
in association with Methuen, Inc.
733 Third Avenue, New York, NY 10017

Typeset in Great Britain by
Scarborough Typesetting Services
and printed in Great Britain by
Richard Clay (The Chaucer Press) Ltd, Bungay, Suffolk

British Library Cataloguing in Publication Data

Social skills and health
1. Group relations training
I. Argyle, Michael
305   HM108

ISBN 0-416-72980-0
ISBN 0-416-72990-8 Pbk

Contents

Notes on the contributors

Michael Argyle is a Fellow of Wolfson College, Oxford and Reader in Social Psychology in the Department of Experimental Psychology, University of Oxford. He is the author of numerous books and articles on social psychology, interpersonal relations and social skills.

Bryn Davis is a trained general and psychiatric nurse. An interest in interpersonal relationships and communication with special reference to student nurse training developed after further training as a nurse tutor, and led to a degree in psychology at Birkbeck College. This was followed by the award of a DHSS Nursing Research Fellowship for postgraduate research at the London School of Economics. Mr Davis has been Deputy Director of the Nursing Research Unit, Department of Nursing Studies at the University of Edinburgh since 1976.

Windy Dryden is a Counselling Psychologist and Lecturer in Education in the Department of Educational Enquiry, University of Aston. He is an Associate Fellow of the Institute for Rational Emotive Therapy, New York, and in addition is on the Institute for RET's training faculty. His principal interests include cognitive aspects of counselling and psychotherapy, therapy with working class patients, and applying social psychological concepts to counselling and psychotherapy.

Barbara L. Hudson is Lecturer in Applied Social Studies (Social Work) at the University of Oxford. She was previously Lecturer in Social Work Studies at the London School of Economics. She trained in social work at the Universities of Chicago and Newcastle upon Tyne, and prior to entering teaching was a Psychiatric Social Worker at St Olave's Hospital (Guy's Group). She is co-editor, with Brian Sheldon, of the *International Journal of Behavioural Social Work & Abstracts*, and has written a book to be published by the Macmillan Press, *Social Work with Psychiatric Patients*.

Peter Maguire is currently a Senior Lecturer in Psychiatry in the University of Manchester and Consultant Psychiatrist to the University Hospital of South Manchester. He is particularly interested in the psychiatric problems which occur in patients with serious physical illness, especially malignant disease. He is also actively involved in helping develop and evaluate different methods of training medical students, doctors and nurses to improve their skills in communicating with patients and their recognition of psychiatric problems in physically ill patients and their relatives.

Myrna Shure is Professor in the Department of Mental Health Sciences, Hahnemann Medical College, Philadelphia, Pennsylvania, USA. In 1966, she received her PhD in Child Development and Family Relationships from Cornell University, Ithaca, New York. Myrna Shure has developed and conducted interpersonal cognitive problem solving programmes for use by parents and teachers of four- and five-year-old children, as well as tests and measures to evaluate those programmes. In addition, she has co-authored three books, and written a series of articles, programmes and testing manuals. She was also principal investigator for a study of problem solving and behaviour in ten-year-olds, funded by the National Institute of Mental Health. Research and training of four- and five-year-olds was supported by Grant #20372, National Institute of Mental Health, 1971–5. The author expresses recognition and sincere appreciation to Bertram Snead, director; Rosemary Mazzatenta, assistant director and Vivian Ray, chief psychologist of the Philadelphia Get Set Day Care, whose receptivity to providing new programmes paved the way for our preventive mental health efforts.

Peter Trower is Senior Clinical Psychologist at Hollymoor Hospital, Northfield, Birmingham. His principal interest is in the various applications of social skills training and he has published a number of books and journal articles on the topic.

Acknowledgements

The editor and publishers would like to thank the following for kind permission to reproduce copyright material:

Penguin Books Ltd for Figure 1.1; University of Chicago Press for Figure 1.2; The British Psychological Society for Figure 1.3; John Wiley & Sons for Figure 1.4.

Introduction

MICHAEL ARGYLE

By 'social skills' we mean the styles of social behaviour used by interviewers, nurses or others in dealing with their clients. As with motor
skills — like skiing, typing or driving a car — some people are more
skilled than others; they are more effective in attaining the required
goals. To study social skills, the effectiveness of different performers
must somehow be measured or assessed. Sometimes there are
objective indices of success, as in the case of selling; sometimes it is
necessary to resort to ratings by supervisors or colleagues. The second
step is to compare the styles of social behaviour used by effective and
ineffective performers of the skill to discover what they do differently
and eventually to define the optimum style of social performance.
The adoption of different social skills can have a considerable effect
on the attainment of goals. The differences in effectiveness between
good and bad performers, or between those at different ends of skills
dimensions, are quite often fivefold in terms of measurable goals, e.g.
the amount sold by salesmen. At the lower end of the scale, performance can be completely useless: supervisors of groups who produce
nothing, psychotherapists whose patients get no better (or get worse),
and selection interviewers whose selections are no better than chance.
These are all jobs where social performance is of crucial importance;
there are plenty of other jobs where it is much less so, such as research
and technical positions, though here too it is necessary to be able to
communicate and co-operate with other people.

When the optimum social skill has been discovered it can then be
taught to trainees on training courses. An implication of the social
skills approach is that specific styles of social behaviour will be taught
— as opposed to attempts at increasing general sensitivity or insight,

as in some other approaches to the problem. In the early stages of social skills training and research emphasis was placed on the correct amount of use of elements of behaviour such as smiling, gaze, head-nods, etc. — and socially inadequate people do make less use of these non-verbal (NV) signals or use them in the wrong way (Trower 1980). Emphasis has been placed on NV signals, since they are important and since trainees are often unaware of the NV signals they are sending, or which are being sent by others. However, verbal behaviour is also highly important, and training can be given for this also.

Awareness of the importance of social skills is fairly recent. The first skill to be studied was probably the supervision of working groups. During the early 1950s, field studies by research workers at the University of Michigan and elsewhere showed some aspects of the most effective style of supervision (Likert 1961). These studies were extensively replicated in several parts of the world and were rapidly incorporated in training courses (Argyle 1980). More details of these skills are given in Argyle (ed.) 1981, Chapter 5. At first such courses used the lecture and discussion method, but this was soon found to be ineffective, and was replaced by more powerful training methods (see Chapter 8). The result must surely be that supervisory skills have been changed throughout much of the western world.

The skills of teaching were discovered at a rather later date, but have been if anything even more widely promoted than supervisory skills (Dunkin and Biddle 1974). We have decided to omit them from this book because of the extensive literature on the subject. Some of the other skills discussed have been studied more recently, and some of them need a good deal more investigation. For example, doctor–patient skills are still not taught in some British medical schools, though nearly all those in America do so. Parent skills are as yet taught on a very limited scale, and here too more research is clearly needed.

While knowledge of particular social skills was developing, intensive laboratory research was being conducted into the basic processes of social interaction of which skilled performance consists. Research at Oxford in the early 1960s into social interaction led to the formulation of the social skill model, which draws on the similarities between social behaviour and the performance of motor skills (Argyle and Kendon 1967). Later research on social interaction at Oxford and elsewhere elaborated that model — for example, by showing the importance of non-verbal signals (Argyle 1975). Some of this research is quite recent − e.g. into sequences of interaction and the analysis of social situations − and it has not yet been fully used by those engaged in the study and teaching of specific skills. Research in other areas, such as the analysis of social relationships, is newer still and has scarcely been applied at all. Research in the applied field, however, often makes fundamental contributions to our knowledge of skills. For example, research on sequences of interaction in the classroom (Flanders 1970, and others) has made an important contribution to the study of sequences of behaviour. These processes are described in Chapter 1.

This volume is about social skills in relation to health. Social skills are very important for nurses, doctors, psychotherapists and social workers; indeed much of their work consists of social performance in relation to patients. Although social skills are of central importance for all these professions, they are not the *only* kind of skill needed; doctors and nurses must know about medicine. The relative import-ance of social skills and technical skills and knowledge varies widely, but the importance of social skills has been greatly underestimated. The social skills of patients themselves are also important, and the contribution of poor social skills to mental disorder is discussed in Chapter 7.

Social skills training (SST) for patients and for other kinds of clients, especially in the USA, has often taken the form of assertiveness training (Rich and Schroeder 1976). However, it must be pointed out that the skills used in making friends and influencing people are quite different. Many socially skilled tasks require forms of influence which have nothing to do with assertiveness. Further, there are cultural differences in the extent to which assertiveness is valued.

Argyle (ed.) 1981 is about social skills and work, and includes several topics which are relevant to health workers, especially those in supervisory or management positions. There are chapters on the skills of supervision, interviewing and negotiation, and there is also a chapter on the skills of inter-cultural communication.

An important problem in using all social skills is the need to vary social behaviour for different clients and in different situations. Research in several areas has shown how skills should vary in this way, and basic research in dyadic interaction has shown how to control the behaviour of others, in interviews or other settings. Recent research into the properties of social situations has shown how skill needs to vary with the social setting. Patterns of social behaviour also vary with class and culture; readers are referred to Argyle (ed.) 1981, Chapter 7 discusses the skills of coping effectively in another culture.

The social skills which are needed in jobs and elsewhere in society are different at different times and places. The same job may have to be done in different ways as the result of technological or other social changes. The power of industrial supervisors is reduced by the extension of industrial democracy and was much greater before the appearance of trade unions. There may be changes in the law which affect the power and responsibilities of social workers and others. Selection interviewers have a different relation to candidates depending on whether jobs are scarce or good applicants are scarce. There have been general changes in social relationships so that a less hierarchical and less authoritarian style of behaviour is now expected in most organizations.

Social changes also create new social roles, which require new social skills. Technological changes have created the roles associated with television, e.g. anchor men, political interviewers and performers at chat shows; other technological changes have led to the appearance of air hostesses — a role that was deliberately created, and for which training is given.

The activities of psychologists led to the roles of psychotherapist, T-group leader and social skills trainer. Now that we know more about social skills, the social skills requirements of new organizational structures should be remembered so that new roles can be carefully designed and appropriate training given.

The use of SST has grown very rapidly during recent years — e.g. for mental patients, prisoners, teachers, managers and doctors — though it has not yet become easily available to the general public. Early forms of training, by lecture and discussion, were soon found to be ineffective, and were replaced by role playing, usually with videotape playback. There have been many follow-up studies of SST, and we can now specify in some detail the form the training should take. These findings are reviewed in Chapter 8. Curiously, those responsible for administering training, in industry and Government for example, have been rather uncritical, have not made greater demands for follow-up studies before commissioning training schemes, and have sometimes approved unsatisfactory forms of training.

The rapid growth of SST has sometimes led to a low-grade, watered-down form of training consisting of rather amateurish role playing. SST is a sophisticated affair and will be successful only if full use is made of knowledge of the skills to be taught and of the best techniques of teaching them. Clearly, however, social skills are not the whole story: in addition to the technical knowledge and skills needed, certain kinds of 'personal growth' are needed for those who are going to hold responsible jobs and make difficult decisions.

Several criticisms have been made of the social skills approach. It is sometimes said that leaders are born and not made, and similar remarks are made of other social skills. Whether there is any *genetic* component of social competence is not known; certainly by the age of 20 some people are very much more socially competent than others, but this is probably from informal, unplanned and chance social learning experiences. However, people can undoubtedly be trained to be more effective performers of social skills, though everyone probably has limits to what he can be trained to do. The same is true of motor skills like performance at sport, though the limiting factors here are chiefly muscular strength and other aspects of physique.

It may be said that a person's effectiveness depends on his power, or other favourable and unfavourable aspects of his situation. These factors are obviously very important, but unfavourable situations can be coped with by using appropriate skills. Fiedler's research (1967) has suggested that a leader whose group does not accept his authority should resort to a different style of supervision. There may be *role conflicts* if conflicting demands are made by other people; doctors, for example, may experience a conflict between looking after their patients and participating in research trials. These require special skills of role bargaining to keep both parties happy. In some roles a number of different people with different points of view must be dealt with; these may be difficult to reconcile, as for social workers who have to deal with the police, doctors, teachers and parents, as well as with their clients.

It is often said that training people in social behaviour encourages deception: pretending to have attitudes and feelings which are not truly felt. Part of the answer is that the rules in some situations and the rules governing a number of professional roles require people to control not only their behaviour but also their emotional states and their attitudes to other people. This can be done by controlling the expression of emotion and by controlling other bodily states, e.g. by relaxation, and control of thoughts and images (Hochschild 1979). Even if such control of feelings and attitudes is unsuccessful it can be argued that teachers, doctors and others should still treat well, i.e. give the appearance of liking, those clients whom they do not like. There is some evidence that real feelings change to fit those which are expressed (Laird 1974).

Another objection to the social skills approach is that people may be made self-conscious by being instructed in the details of social performance. The experience of trainers is that this is only a temporary phenomenon; after the second training session most trainees focus their attention once again on the job in hand and the behaviour of the others present rather than on their own performance. Finally it is sometimes objected that the use of skilled social techniques is a form of 'manipulation' of others. This is a curious point: if a teacher teaches effectively, or a doctor cures patients, this would not be regarded as manipulation, which presumably refers to successful social influence of a kind which is thought socially undesirable. Perhaps the use of subtle, or non-verbal, social skills is regarded with more suspicion than the use of more obvious, or verbal, skills. The social skills approach extends the range of social techniques beyond those which are familiar. It must be hoped that the new skills will be used more for desirable social ends than for undesirable ones.

References

Argyle, M. (1975). *Bodily Communication*. London: Methuen.

_____ (1980). The development of applied social psychology. *In* Gilmour, R. and Duck, S. (eds). *The Development of Social Psychology*. London: Academic Press, pp. 81–105.

Argyle, M. (ed.) (1981) *Social Skills and Work*. London: Methuen.

Argyle, M. and Kendon, A. (1967). The experimental analysis of social performance. *In* Berkowitz, L. (ed.). *Advances in Experimental Social Psychology*. New York: Academic Press, vol. 3, pp. 55–98.

Dunkin, M. J. and Biddle, B. J. (1974). *The Study of Teaching*. New York: Holt, Rinehart and Winston.

Fiedler, F. E. (1967). *A Theory of Leadership Effectiveness*. New York: McGraw-Hill.

Flanders, N. A. (1970). *Analyzing Teaching Behavior*. Reading, Mass.: Addison-Wesley.

Hochschild, A. R. (1979). Emotion work, feeling rules and social structures. *Am. J. Sociol* 85, 551–75.

Laird, J. D. (1974). Self-attribution of emotion: the effects of expressive behavior on the quality of emotional experience. *J. Pers. Soc. Psychol.* 29, 475–86.

Likert, R. (1961). *New Patterns of Management*. New York: McGraw-Hill.

Rich, A. P. and Schroeder, H. E. (1976). Research issues in assertiveness training. *Psychol. Bull.* 83, 1081–96.

Trower, P. (1980). Situational analysis of the components and processes of behavior of socially skilled and unskilled patients. *J. Consult. Clin. Psychol.* 48, 327–39.

1 The nature of social skill

MICHAEL ARGYLE

Introduction

By socially skilled behaviour I mean social behaviour which is effective in realizing the goals of the interactor. These may be the professional goals of doctors, nurses and social workers, or of various kinds of interviewers, supervisors, chairmen, etc. as discussed in this book. In most of the chapters in this book the goals of particular skills are described. In some cases there are several different goals, which are not always compatible with each other. The goals may also include the personal goals of wanting to make friends and influence people in everyday life.

By comparing the styles of social behaviour of effective and ineffective performers it is possible to discover the kinds of social behaviour which lead to the desired results in particular settings, and thus constitute socially skilled behaviour. Many examples of such research, and of the styles of social behaviour shown to be most effective, will be given in later chapters. The effects of different styles of performance in attaining goals can be very great. Early research on supervisory skills, for example, found that supervisors who scored high in certain dimensions of supervisory skill produced one-fifth of the absenteeism and labour turnover of those low in such dimensions.

In this chapter I shall try to set out the main results of research into the basic processes used in skilled behaviour. This can open up new areas of research into more practical aspects of social competence. For example, research on the properties of interaction sequences may suggest new ways of looking at the behaviour of effective and ineffective performers, and hence at aspects of behaviour which could be made the focus of training. Examples are failures to handle conversational sequences and the structuring of such sequences by skilled performers (p. 173).

The social skill model

This model draws attention to a number of analogies between social performance and the performance of motor skills like driving a car (see Fig. 1.1). In each case the performer pursues certain goals, makes continuous response to feedback and emits hierarchically-organized motor responses. This model has been heuristically very useful in drawing attention to the importance of feedback, and hence to gaze; it also suggests a number of different ways in which social performances can fail and the training procedures that may be effective, through analogy with motor skills training (Argyle and Kendon 1967, Argyle 1969).

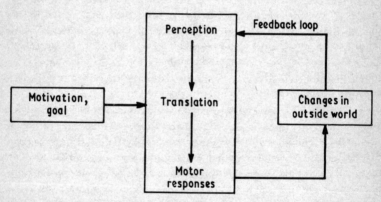

Figure 1.1   The social skill model (from Argyle 1967).

The model emphasizes the motivation, goals and plans of inter-actors. It is postulated that every interactor is trying to achieve some goal, whether he is aware of it or not. These goals may be to get another person to like him, to obtain or convey information, to modify the other's emotional state, and so on. Such goals may be linked to more basic motivational systems. Goals have sub-goals: for example a doctor must diagnose the patient's disease before he can treat him. Patterns of response are directed towards goals and sub-goals, and have a hierarchical structure — large units of behaviour are composed of smaller ones, and at the lowest levels these are habitual and automatic.

Harré and Secord (1972) have argued persuasively that much human social behaviour is the result of conscious planning, often in words, with full regard for the complex meanings of behaviour and the rules of situations. This is an important correction to earlier social psychological views, which often failed to recognize the complexity of individual planning and the different meanings which may be given to stimuli, for example in laboratory experiments. However, it must be recognized that much social behaviour is *not* planned in this way: the smaller elements of behaviour and longer automatic sequences are outside conscious awareness — though it is possible to attend, for example, to patterns of gaze, shifts of orientation or the latent meanings of utterances. The social skills model, in emphasizing the hierarchical structure of social performance, can incorporate both kinds of behaviour. There is another important implication of this line of thought: the moves, or social acts, made in social behaviour are rather different from the actions in a motor skill. Social acts, like shaking hands, bidding at an auction sale or asking questions at a seminar are signals with a shared social meaning in a given context. They are like the moves in a game: in any particular game there is a repertoire of possible moves, which is quite different for chess, polo or wrestling; each move has a generally accepted meaning in the context of the game and the move can be made by alternative physical actions.

The social skill model also emphasizes feedback processes. A person driving a car sees at once when it is going in the wrong direction, and takes corrective action with the steering wheel. Social interactors do likewise; if another person is talking too much they interrupt, ask closed questions or no questions and look less interested in what he has to say. Feedback requires perception, looking at and listening to the other person. Skilled performance requires the ability to take the appropriate corrective action referred to as 'translation' in the model — not everyone knows that open-ended questions make people talk more and closed questions make them talk less. It also depends on a number of two-step sequences of social behaviour whereby certain social acts have reliable effects on another. The social skills which are most effective vary with the situation, and also with culture and social class. Cultural differences in social behaviour are described in

Argyle (ed.) (1981). Shure (Chapter 6) describes how to train people in a problem-solving approach to difficult social situations, whereby they are encouraged to engage in 'means—ends thinking'. Maladjusted adolescents were less able than controls to formulate a step-by-step plan to deal with situations. In the selection interview various kinds of difficult candidates must be dealt with and interviewers can be taught the special skills needed for each. The 'translation' part of the model often includes complex cognitive structures, including the rules and other features of the immediate situation and knowledge of social processes (Pendleton and Furnham 1980).

It is an interactor's *behaviour* which affects other people, but the model also applies to the control of thought and feelings. Hochschild (1979) has argued that social skills performers, especially those in professional roles, are expected to have the right feelings — to be happy, sad, grateful, etc. where appropriate.

The role of reinforcement

This is one of the key processes in social skill sequences. When interactor A does what B wants him to do, B is pleased and sends immediate and spontaneous reinforcements — smile, gaze, approving noises, etc. — and modifies A's behaviour, probably by operant conditioning, for example by modifying the content of A's utterances (Rosenfeld 1978). At the same time A is modifying B's behaviour in exactly the same way. These effects appear to be mainly outside the focus of conscious attention and take place very rapidly. It follows that anyone who gives strong rewards and punishments in the course of interaction will be able to modify the behaviour of others in the desired direction. In addition, the stronger the rewards that A issues, the more strongly other people will be attracted to him.

The role of gaze in social skills

The social skill model suggests that the monitoring of another's reactions is an essential part of social performance. The other's verbal signals are mainly heard, but his non-verbal (NV) signals are mainly seen — the exceptions being the NV aspects of speech and touch. It was this implication of the social skill model which directed the study of gaze in social interaction. In dyadic interaction each person looks about 50 per cent of the time, mutual gaze occupies 25 per cent of the time, looking while listening occurs about twice as long as looking while talking, glances are about 3 seconds, and mutual glances about 21 seconds, with wide variations due to distance, sex combinations and personality (Argyle and Cook 1976).

Differences between social behaviour and motor skills

Rules   The moves which interactors may make are governed by rules; they must respond properly to what has gone before. Similarly, rules govern the other's responses and can be used to influence his behaviour, e.g. questions lead to answers.

Taking the role of the other   It is important to perceive accurately the reactions of others, and the perceptions of others − i.e. their point of view − must also be perceived. This appears to be a cognitive ability which develops with age (Flavell 1968), but which may fail to develop properly. Those who are able to do this have been found to be more effective at a number of social tasks and more altruistic. Shure (Chapter 6) describes how to train parents and children in recognizing the points of view of other people in difficult situations.

The independent initiative of others   Other interactors are also pursuing *their* goals, reacting to feedback and so on. The social skills model itself deals with one interactor at a time; to deal with sequences of social interaction further concepts must be introduced. I shall discuss below the ways of analysing these sequences of interaction. The social skill model fits best cases of 'asymmetrical contingency' (interviewing, teaching, etc.), where one person is more or less in charge. In such cases the social skills used by effective and less effective performers may be compared. On the other hand, in negotiation both sides have a similar degree of initiative.

The psychology of the other   While cars and typewriters behave in accordance with physical laws, persons and groups follow psychological laws. To be able to handle them effectively it helps to have some understanding of the processes used. For example, when using presenting skills the psychology of attention and memory is important. For the skills of supervision the social psychology of groups is needed.

Verbal communication

When the behaviour of successful and less successful performers of a skill is compared, aspects of verbal communication are often found to be important. Trower (1980) found that the sheer amount of verbal output was the main difference between socially skilled and unskilled patients; Romano and Bellack (1980) found that offering alternatives and reasons were the best predictors of assertiveness; studies of teachers, supervisors and others have found the specific aspects of verbal performance which are most important.

Different kinds of utterance

There are several different kinds of verbal utterance:

Egocentric speech   This is directed to the self and is found in infants and has the effect of directing behaviour.

Orders and instructions   These are used to influence the behaviour of others; they can be gently persuasive or authoritarian.

Questions   These are intended to elicit verbal information; they can be open-ended or closed, personal or impersonal.

Information   This may be given in response to a question, or part of a lecture, or during a problem-solving discussion.

The last three above are the basic classes of utterance.

Informal speech   This consists of casual chat, jokes and gossip and contains little information, but helps to establish and sustain social relationships.

Expression of emotions and interpersonal attitudes   This is a special kind of information; however, this information is usually conveyed, and is conveyed more effectively, non-verbally.

'Performative' utterances   These include 'illocutions' where saying the utterance performs something (voting, judging, naming, etc.) and 'perlocutions', where a goal is intended but may not be achieved (persuading, intimidating, etc.).

Social routines These include standard sequences like thanking, apologizing, greeting, etc.

Latent messages These are where the more important meaning is made subordinate: 'As I was saying to the Prime Minister'.

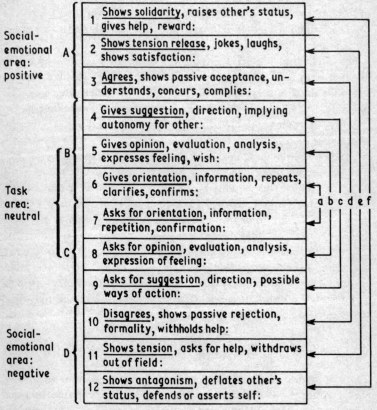

Key
a Problems of communication   b Problems of evaluation
c Problems of control   d Problems of decision
e Problems of tension reduction   f Problems of reintegration
A Positive reactions   B Attempted answers
C Questions   D Negative reactions

Figure 1.2   The Bales categories (from Bales 1950).

There are many category schemes for reducing utterances to a limited number of classes of social acts. One of the best known is that of Bales (1950), who introduced the twelve classes shown in Figure 1.2.

Although such schemes have been widely used, there is a fundamental difficulty in using them in that the same utterance may need
to be classified in several different ways for different purposes. A discussion may include a large number of questions and suggestions, but
they are *different* questions, and it would not be possible to trace the
argument by Bales analysis alone. The same utterance may be a
question which is open-ended, rude and long; each feature may affect
some aspect of the response.

For each kind of social situation a different set of categories is
needed, both for analysing what is happening and to train people in
the skills used. For example, in negotiation a repertoire of special
moves is used which is rather different from the repertoire for psychotherapy (Chapter 4), or children at play, or interaction in the family
(Argyle, *et al.* 1981).

Utterances follow each other in a conversation in special ways. The
meaning of an utterance may depend on other utterances (e.g. 'I
disagree'), or on the social setting ('Forty–love'), and it may not be
what it seems: 'Could you pass the salt?' is usually not a question; 'Come
in' may not be an order but a welcome. A speaker usually produces
utterances that he thinks the hearer can understand, and he adjusts its
technicality and the use of local references. Encoding anticipates
decoding. Rommetveit (1974) has show how each utterance takes
account of the shared information and objects of attention of speaker
and hearer and adds to them. The new is nested in the old. The
structure of sequences of utterance will now be discussed.

Non-verbal signals accompanying speech

Completing and elaborating on verbal utterances   Some utterances
are meaningless or ambiguous unless the NV accompaniments are
taken into account. A lecturer may point at part of a diagram: a tape-
recording of this part of the lecture would be meaningless. Some
sentences are ambiguous if printed conventionally – 'They are
hunting dogs' – but not if spoken – 'They are hunting *dogs*'.
Gestural illustrations are used to amplify the meaning of utterances,
and succeed in doing so. The way in which an utterance is delivered
'frames' it, i.e. the intonation and facial expression indicate whether
it is intended to be serious, funny, sarcastic (implying the opposite),
rhetorical or requiring an answer and so on; the NV accompaniment
is a message about the message, which is needed by the recipient to

know what to do with it. There are finer comments and elaborations: particular words can be given emphasis, pronounced in a special accent, or in a way suggesting a particular attitude. The most important NV signals here are the prosodic aspects of vocalization — the timing, pitch and loudness of speech. The gestural accompaniments of speech are also important, particularly illustrators. Facial expression and glances accompany speech in a similar way. The importance of tone of voice is discussed in Chapter 4 on psychotherapy.

Managing synchronizing When two or more people are talking they have to take turns to speak. This is achieved mainly by using NV signals. For example, if a speaker wants to avoid being interrupted he will be more successful if he does not look up at the ends of sentences, keeps a hand in mid-gesture at these points, and if he immediately increases the loudness of his speech when interrupted. Kendon (1967) showed that a speaker can hand over the conversation smoothly to another speaker by asking a question and giving a terminal gaze. However, Beattie (1980) found that questions were asked at only 22.5 per cent of smooth switches, and that terminal gaze made a difference only if it occurred during a period of hesitant speech with a low amount of gaze. Duncan and Fiske (1977) found that six different signals were associated with turn-taking; in a replication Beattie found that the strongest signals were clause completion and change in pitch level. However, at 20 per cent of smooth switches none of these signals were present — so some of the art of synchronizing is yet to be discovered.

Sending feedback signals When someone is speaking he needs intermittent but regular feedback on how others are responding so that he can modify his utterances accordingly. He needs to know whether the listeners understand, believe or disbelieve, are surprised or bored, agree or disagree, are pleased or annoyed. This information could be provided by *sotto voce* verbal muttering on their part, but is in fact obtained by careful study of the listener's face: the eyebrows signal surprise, puzzlement, etc.; while the mouth indicates pleasure and displeasure. When the other is invisible, as in telephone conversation, these visual signals are unavailable, and more verbalized 'listening behaviour' is used — 'I see', 'Really?', 'How interesting', etc.

Speech styles

People use different speech styles in different situations. On informal occasions they use informal speech, which is characterized by simpler structure of sentences, less accurate grammar, more verbs and pronouns, fewer nouns and adjectives and more slang.

Speech can be delivered in different accents, with different speeds, loudness and emotional tones, all of which govern the social effect of an utterance. Emotional tone is conveyed by various physical parameters; depression, for example, is conveyed by slow speed, low pitch and low volume. Accent consists of the ways in which various phonemes are pronounced, e.g. making 'a' long or short, and conveys information about social class, education and regional origins. Research by Lambert and Giles has shown that if the same speaker makes several recordings in different accents, he is perceived and evaluated quite differently; for example, stereotyped judgments about English and French Canadians would be expressed. When people who normally use different speech styles interact they usually converge towards a similar manner of speaking, probably to increase social acceptance by each other (Giles and Powesland 1975).

Non-verbal communication (NVC)

When successful and less successful performers of a skill are compared, NVC is always found to be an important area of difference. Trower (1980) found that socially skilled patients looked, smiled and gestured more than unskilled ones. Romano and Bellack (1980) found that ratings on assertiveness were predictable from smiling and vocal intonation. NVC consists of facial expression, tone of voice, gaze, gestures, postures, physical proximity and appearance. We have already described how NVC is linked with speech; it also functions in several other ways, especially in the communication of emotions and attitudes to other people.

A *sender* is in a certain state, or possesses some information; this is *encoded* into a message which is then *decoded* by a *receiver*:

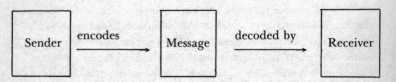

Encoding research is done by putting subjects into some state and studying the NV messages which are emitted. For example, Mehrabian (1971) asked subjects in a role-playing experiment to address a hatstand, imagining it to be a person. Male subjects who liked the hatstand looked at it more, did not have hands on hips and stood closer.

Decoding research is done by presenting experimentally prepared stimuli to subjects and finding how they are decoded. Argyle, Lefebvre and Cook (1974) taught confederates five patterns of gaze, which they used with different subjects, who gave their impressions of the confederates in the form of ratings. The main result was that the confederates were liked more if they looked more, unless they looked more than the spontaneous rate, though ratings on scales of activity and dominance increased continuously with their level of gaze.

The meaning of a non-verbal signal can be given in terms of how it is encoded or decoded. These meanings are of two main kinds. Signals may be analogical, as with gestures similar to the object described and some facial expressions − e.g. showing the teeth by animals, which is part of an act of biting. Or signals can have arbitrary meanings as the result of past associations, as with clothes, hair styles or conventional gestures. NV signals may have meanings which are not readily expressed in words. There are research methods for finding such meanings, such as multidimensional scaling, in which subjects are asked to rate the similarity between photographs of facial expressions; this generates dimensions defined only in terms of the photographs. Some NV signals appear to have no subjective meaning at all, though they do influence behaviour − as in the case of small head-nods or shifts of gaze. Such signals may be said to have a behavioural meaning. Similar considerations may be applied to some ritual signals like handshakes, which accomplish a change of relationship but have no obvious subjective meaning.

Non-verbal signals are often 'unconscious', i.e. are outside the focus of attention. A few signals are unconsciously sent and received, like dilated pupils signifying sexual attraction, but there are a number of other possibilities, as shown in Table 1.1. Strictly speaking pupil dilation is not communication at all, but only a physiological response. 'Communication' is usually taken to imply some intention to affect another person; one criterion is that it makes a difference whether the other person is present and in a position to receive the signal; another is that the signal is repeated, varied or amplified if it

Table 1.1   Awareness of non-verbal signals

Awareness of:		Factor governing awareness
Sender	*Receiver*	
Aware	Aware	Verbal signal
Mostly unaware	Mostly aware	Most NVC
Aware	Unaware	Trained sender
Unaware	Aware	Trained receiver
Unaware	Unaware	Some NVC

has no effect. These criteria are independent of conscious intention to communicate, which is often absent.

The functions of NVC

Interpersonal attitudes   This section deals with attitudes towards others who are present. The main attitudes fall along two dimensions:

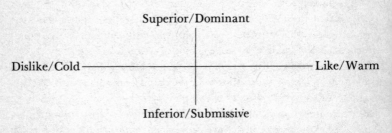

In addition there is love, which is a variant of like. These attitudes can be conveyed clearly by NV signals, such as facial expression, tone of voice and posture. Liking is conveyed by smiling, a friendly tone of voice and so on.

These NV cues combine together to signal, for example, the overall degree of liking felt by an interactor. Between two people NV signals reflect the degree of intimacy between them. Argyle and Dean (1965) showed that gaze and distance vary inversely, and suggested more generally that the different cues for intimacy — smiling, tone of voice, leaning forwards, etc. — can be substituted for each other. There has been a good deal of support for this theory (Patterson 1973), but a positive NV signal can lead to reciprocation (rather than to equilibration) — up to a point — if it is interpreted as clearly positive (Patterson 1976).

I and my colleagues compared the effect of verbal and non-verbal signals for communicating interpersonal attitudes. Typed messages were prepared indicating that the speaking was superior, equal or inferior; videotapes of a performer counting (1, 2, 3 . . .) were made, conveying the same attitudes; the verbal and non-verbal signals were rated by subjects as very similar in superiority, etc. The nine combined signals were presented to further subjects on videotape − superior (verbal), inferior (non-verbal), etc. − and rated for superiority. The variance due to NV cues was about twelve times the variance due to verbal cues in affecting judgments of inferior−superior (Argyle, *et al.* 1970). Some of the results are shown in Figure 1.3. Similar results were obtained in later experiments with friendly−hostile messages (Argyle, *et al.* 1972).

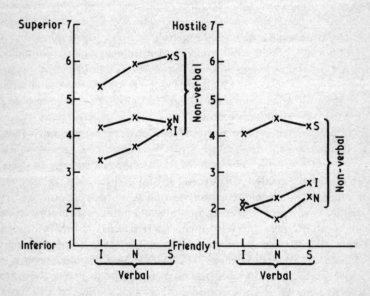

Figure 1.3   Effects of inferior, neutral and superior verbal and non-verbal signals on semantic rating (from Argyle *et al.* 1970).

The attitudes of others are perceived, then, mainly from their non-verbal behaviour. People can judge with some accuracy when others like them, but are much less accurate in perceiving dislike (Tagiuri 1958). The reason for this is probably that expressions of dislike are concealed to a large extent and only the more subtle ones remain, such as bodily orientation.

Emotional states   These can be distinguished from interpersonal attitudes in that emotions are not directed towards others present but are simply states of the individual. The common emotions are anger, depression, anxiety, joy, surprise, fear and disgust/contempt (Ekman, *et al.* 1972). An anxious state, for example, can be shown by: (a) *tone of voice* − breathy, rapid, speech errors; (b) *facial expression* − tense, perspiring, expanded pupils; (c) *posture* − tense and rigid; (d) *gestures* − tense clasping of objects, or general bodily activity; (e) *smell* − of perspiration; and (f) *gaze* − short glances, aversion of gaze. Interactors may try to conceal their true emotional state, or to convey that they are in some different emotional condition, but it is difficult to control all of these cues, and impossible to control more autonomic ones. Emotional states can be conveyed by speech − 'I am feeling very happy' − but such statements will not be believed unless supported by appropriate NVC, and the NVC can convey the message without the speech.

There are considerable individual differences in the extent to which emotions are expressed. Buck (1979) has shown that there are 'internalizers', who have high physiological arousal during emotion but little facial expression, and 'externalizers' who do the opposite; females tend to be externalizers.

I have focused so far mainly on facial expression and tone of voice, since these are the most important NV signals for interpersonal attitudes and emotions. There are several other NV signals, however, which are of considerable interest. Spatial position − proximity and orientation − also express interpersonal attitudes, such as friendly−hostile, and co-operative−competitive. Gestures are used in conjunction with speech to supplement and replace it, especially for ideas which are hard to put into words; the Italians have a large vocabulary of gestures with definite meanings. Clothes, hair and other aspects of appearance are used in self-presentation to send messages about the self (Argyle 1975).

Other functions of NVC   NVC accompanies speech, as we have seen (p. 8). It is the main channel for self-presentation (p. 26), and plays an important part in rituals.

The perception of other people

To respond effectively to the behaviour of others it is necessary to perceive them correctly. The social skill model emphasizes the importance of perception and feedback: to drive a car one must watch the traffic outside and the instruments inside. Such perception consists of selecting certain cues, and being able to interpret them correctly. This selection and interpretation can lead to serious errors, especially for mental patients (see p. 172). Professional social skill performers must select relevant aspects of other people's behaviour and interpret it in terms of categories appropriate to the skill. For example doctors may attend to the skin condition and other aspects of their client's body and interpret such cues in terms of health and disease; however, these are not the most important cues for negotiators or salesmen to attend to. In addition to forming impressions of other people, interactors need to perceive others' emotional states and attitudes to the interactor, and to be fully aware of the moment-to-moment development of encounters. For selection interviewers and clinical psychologists the appraisal of others is a central part of the job.

We form impressions of other people all the time, mainly to predict their future behaviour, and so that we can deal with them effectively. We categorize others in terms of our favourite cognitive constructs, of which the most widely used are:

Extraversion, sociability.
Agreeableness, likeability.
Emotional stability.
Intelligence.
Assertiveness.

There are, however, wide individual differences in the constructs used, and 'complex' people use a larger number of such dimensions. We have found that the constructs used vary greatly with the situation; for example, work-related constructs are not used in purely social situations. We also found that the constructs used vary with the target group, e.g. children *v.* psychologists (Argyle, *et al.* 1981).

There are a number of widespread errors in forming impressions of others, which should particularly be avoided by those whose job it is to assess others:

(a) Assuming that a person's behaviour is mainly a product of his personality, whereas it may be more a function of the situation he is in: at a noisy party, in church, etc.
(b) Assuming that his behaviour is due to him rather than his role, e.g. as a hospital nurse *v.* patient *v.* visitor.

(c) Placing too much importance on physical cues, like beards, clothes and physical attractiveness.
(d) Being affected by stereotypes about the characteristics of members of certain races, social classes, etc.

The main job of selection interviewers (Volume II, Chapter 1) is to form accurate impressions of candidates, and it is important for them to avoid these and other principal errors.

During social interaction it is also necessary to perceive the emotional state of others; for example, to tell if they are depressed or angry. There are wide individual differences in ability to judge emotions correctly (Davitz 1964). As we have seen, emotions are mainly conveyed by NV signals, especially by facial expression and tone of voice. The interpretation of emotions is also based on perception of the situation the other person is in. M. G. Lalljee at Oxford (unpublished observations) found that smiles are not necessarily decoded as happy, whereas unhappy faces are usually regarded as authentic. Emotional states are often concealed though there may be 'leakage' of the true situation via hands, feet, tone of voice or other channels which are difficult to control. Psychotherapists need to know about the emotions of their clients and thus pay particular attention to such cues (p. 96).

Similar considerations apply to the perception of interpersonal attitudes, e.g. who likes whom, which is also based mainly on NV signals, such as proximity, gaze and facial expression. Again use is made of context to decode these signals — a glance at a stranger may be interpreted as a threat, an appeal for help or a friendly invitation. There are some interesting errors due to pressures towards cognitive consistency: if A likes B, he thinks that B likes him more than B on average actually does; if A likes both B and C, he assumes that they both like each other more than, on average, they do.

It is necessary to perceive the flow of interaction to know what is happening and to participate in it effectively. People seem to agree on the main episodes and sub-episodes of an encounter, but they may produce rather different accounts of why those present behaved as they did. One source of variation, and indeed error, is that people attribute the causes of others' behaviour to their personality — 'She fell over because she is clumsy' — but their own behaviour to the situation — 'I fell over because it was slippery' — whereas both factors operate in each case (Jones and Nisbett 1972). Interpretations also depend on the ideas and knowledge an individual possesses: just as an expert on cars could understand better than a non-expert why a car was behaving in a peculiar way, so an expert on social behaviour could understand why patterns of social behaviour occur.

Sequences of social behaviour

Social behaviour consists of sequences of utterances and NV signals. For such a sequence to constitute an acceptable piece of social behaviour the moves must fit together in order. Social psychologists have not yet discovered all the principles or 'grammar' underlying these sequences but some of the principles are known and can explain common forms of interaction failure.

Two-step sequences

Conversational sequences are constructed partly out of certain basic building blocks, like the question—answer sequence, and repeated cycles characteristic of the situation. Socially inadequate people are usually very bad conversationalists and this appears to be due to a failure to master some of these basic sequences.

There are several other common two-step sequences such as joke—laugh, complain—sympathize, request—comply or refuse. There are a number of two-step sequences which take place not because there is a rule, but as a result of basic psychological processes. For example, there is the powerful effect of reinforcement and there is response-matching, in which one person copies the accent, posture or other aspects of the other's behaviour.

There are also *pro-active* two-step sequences, where one person makes both moves, as in accept—thank, reply—question. Failure to make a pro-active move can stop a conversation.

These reactive and pro-active two-step pairs can build up to make repeated cycles, as happens in the classroom:

```
Teacher  :  lectures
Teacher  :  asks questions
Pupil    :  replies
Teacher  :  comments
(cycle repeats)                        (after Flanders 1970).
```

Social skill sequences

I shall now discuss sequences of more than two steps. The social skill model generates a characteristic kind of four-step sequence:

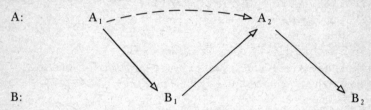

This is a case of asymmetrical interaction with A in charge. A's first move, A_1, produces an unsatisfactory result, B_1, so A modifies his behaviour to A_2, which produces the desired B_2. Note the link A_1-A_2, representing the persistence of A's goal-directed behaviour. This can be seen in the research interview:

I_1: asks questions
R_1: gives inadequate answer, or does not understand question
I_2: clarifies and repeats question
R_2: gives adequate answer

or

I_1: asks question
R_1: refuses to answer
I_2: explains purpose and importance of survey; repeats question
R_2: gives adequate answer

The model can be extended to cases where both interactors are pursuing goals simultaneously, as in the following example, from a selection interview:

I_1: How well did you do at physics at school?
R_1: Not very well, I was better at chemistry.
I_2: What were your A-level results?
R_2: I got a C in physics, and an A in chemistry.
I_3: That's very good.

There are four two-step sequences here: I_1-R_1, I_2-R_2 and R_1-I_2, R_2-I_3. There is persistence and continuity between R_1 and R_2, as well as I_1 and I_2. Although I has the initiative, R can also pursue his goals.

Another set of sequences are the 'social routines' described by

Goffman (1971). An example is the 'remedial sequence': the behaviour which takes place when someone has committed a social error of some kind:

(1) A commits error (e.g. steps on B's toe).
(2) A apologizes, gives excuse or explanation ('I'm frightfully sorry, I didn't see your foot').
(3) B accepts this ('It's OK, no damage done').
(4) A thanks B ('It's very good of you to be so nice about it').
(5) B minimizes what A has done ('Think nothing of it').

Other such routines are those of greeting, opening conversations with strangers, introductions, thanking and parting.

Episode sequences

Most social encounters consist of a number of distinct episodes, which may have to come in a particular order. For example, the doctor–patient interview is said to have six phases, while negotiations have three.

We have found that encounters usually have five main episodes or phases:

(1) Greeting.
(2) Establish relationship.
(3) Central task.
(4) Re-establish relationship.
(5) Parting.

The task in turn may consist of several sub-tasks, e.g. a doctor has to conduct a verbal or physical examination, make a diagnosis and carry out or prescribe treatment. Often, as in this case, the sub-tasks have to come in a certain order. At primarily social events, the 'task' seems to consist of eating or drinking accompanied by the exchange of information.

Situations, their rules and other features

The traditional trait model supposed that individuals possess a fixed degree of introversion, neuroticism, etc., and that it is displayed consistently in different situations. This model has been abandoned by most psychologists because of an increased awareness of the great effect of the situation on behaviour (e.g. people are more anxious when exposed to physical danger than when asleep in bed), and the amount of person–situation interaction (e.g. person A is more frightened by heights, B by cows), resulting in low inter-situational consistency (Mischel 1968).

A long series of studies (Endler and Magnusson 1976) attempted to test trait theory and other models by finding the percentages of variance due to persons (P), situations (S) and P × S interaction. This was done with reported behaviour (e.g. anxiety), and with observed behaviour (e.g. talking, smiling). Typical results were:

Persons	15–30 per cent
Situations	20–45 per cent
P × S	30–50 per cent

(Unfortunately it is not possible to give any exact figures, since there is no way of producing equivalent degrees of variation in personality and situation.) These results show that a simple trait theory must be abandoned. The alternative model which has developed is based on interactionism; this recognizes the independent contribution of persons, situations and interactions between them, and accepts that the detailed prediction of behaviour requires equations of the form $B = f(P, S)$.

However, the interactionist model has a number of serious limitations:

(1) People choose the situations in which they are found, and avoid others, so P has two different effects.
(2) People can to some extent change the situation they are in, for example generating friendly or hostile behaviour from others.
(3) Although some behaviour occurs in all situations, e.g. level of anxiety and amount of talk, situations also have repertoires of behaviour which are unique to them — the moves in chess are different from those in football. The interactionist equations cannot be applied here.
(4) There are problems about specifying the dimensions of situations to enter into the equations, as will be shown below.

Whether we adopt the interactionist position or some other we need to be able to measure or assess situations. Several of the skills which are discussed in this book take place in a variety of different situations. This is particularly true of social work (Chapter 5), selling (Argyle (ed.) 1981, Chapter 3) and supervision (Argyle (ed.) 1981, Chapter 5). In each situation somewhat different skills may be required. One way to classify situations is in terms of the behaviour in them, but this makes it impossible to predict or explain behaviour in terms of properties of situations. Another method is to see how subjects classify situations cognitively, using methods like multi-dimensional scaling. This produces dimensions like formal—informal, friendly—hostile, equal—unequal, task—social, etc. (Wish and Kaplan 1977). This is a good start but doesn't tell us much about the behaviour required in, for example, a selection interview, a confessional, a visit to a psychoanalyst or a judo lesson — all of which are task, friendly and unequal. To do this we have to study the fundamental features of situations (Argyle, Furnham and Graham, 1981). The main features appear to be as follows:

Goals

In all situations there are certain goals which are commonly obtainable. It is often fairly obvious what these are, but socially inadequate people may simply not know what parties are for, for example, or may think that the purpose of a selection interview is vocational guidance.

We have studied the main goals in a number of common situations by asking samples of people to rate the importance of various goals and then carrying out factor analyses. The main goals are usually: (1) social acceptance, etc.; (2) food, drink and other bodily needs; (3) task goals specific to the situation. We have also studied the relations between goals, within and between persons, in terms of conflict and instrumentality. An example of this is given below under 'handling relationships'.

Rules

All situations have rules about what may or may not be done in them. Socially inexperienced people are often ignorant or mistaken about the rules. It would obviously be impossible to play a game without knowing the rules, and the same applies to social situations.

We have studied the rules of a number of everyday situations. There appear to be several universal rules — be polite, be friendly, don't embarrass people. There are also rules which are specific to situations, or groups of situations, and these can be interpreted as functional, since they enable situational goals to be met. For example, when seeing the doctor one should be clean and tell the truth, when going to a party one should dress smartly and keep to cheerful topics of conversation (Argyle, *et al.* 1979).

Special skills

Many social situations require special social skills, as in the various kinds of public speaking and interviewing but also in such everyday situations as dates and parties. A person with little experience of a particular situation may find that he lacks the special skills needed for it (*cf.* Argyle, Furnham and Graham, 1981).

Repertoire of elements

Every situation defines certain moves as relevant. For example, at a seminar it is relevant to show slides, make long speeches, draw on the blackboard, etc. If moves appropriate to a cricket match or a Scottish ball were made, they would be ignored or regarded as totally bizarre. We have found the 65–90 main elements used in several situations, like going to the doctor. We have also found that the semiotic structure varies between situations; questions about work and about private life were sharply contrasted in an office situation, but not on a date.

Roles

Every situation has a limited number of roles, e.g. a classroom has the roles of teacher, pupil, janitor and school inspector. These roles carry different degrees of power, and the occupant has goals peculiar to that role.

Cognitive structure

We found that the members of a research group classified each other in terms of the concepts *extraverted* and *enjoyable companion* for social occasions, but in terms of *dominant*, *creative* and *supportive* for seminars. There are also concepts related to the task, e.g. 'amendment', 'straw vote', 'nem. con.', for committee meetings.

Environmental setting and pieces

Most situations include special environmental settings and props.

Cricket needs bat, ball, stumps, etc.; a seminar usually requires blackboard, slide projector and lecture notes.

How do persons fit into situations, conceived in this way? To begin with, there are certain pervasive aspects of persons, corresponding to the 20 per cent or so of person variance found in P × S studies. This consists of scores on general dimensions like intelligence, extraversion, neuroticism and so on. In addition persons have dispositions to behave in certain ways in classes of situations; this corresponds to the 40 per cent or so of the P × S variance in relation to dimensions of situations like formal–informal, and friendly–hostile. Thirdly there will be more specific reactions to particular situations; for example, behaviour in social psychology seminars will depend partly on knowledge of social psychology, and attitudes to different schools of thought in it. Taken together these three factors may predict avoidance of certain situations – because of lack of skill, anxiety, etc. – which will be the main expectation in such cases.

Handling relationships

All skills require the establishment of a special relationship with the clients, and some require the maintenance of long-term relationships. As with situations, relationships can be classified in various ways. Wish and Kaplan (1977) found the same dimensions for relationships as for situations. From this and other studies it is clear that co-operative (or friendly), and dominant (or assertive) are two dimensions of great importance here.

Establishing a friendly relationship

Research on friendship shows that friends are usually similar – in values, interests and background. Where the social skills performer and a client are dissimilar greater efforts will be needed. Friendship is partly brought about by proximity, e.g. sharing an office, or other sources of frequent interaction. B will like A if he behaves in the following ways:

(1) He should be rewarding – kind, helpful, cheerful, interesting, etc.
(2) He should not be egocentric, but should take a real interest in others.

(3) He should express positive attitudes to others non-verbally, especially by facial expressions and tone of voice.
(4) He should produce appropriate degrees of self-disclosure — gradually increasing, and reciprocating those of the other. Special social moves are needed to make friends — invitations to suitable social events, including drinking, eating, talking or pursuit of joint leisure.

Friendship advances through several stages of increasing intimacy, disclosure and commitment and is sustained by regular encounters, such as meals together, and gifts (Duck 1977).

Establishing a dominant relationship

Often a social skill performer has a position of some power and influence, and the clients accept his authority — as for doctors and selection interviewers. In other cases this is less so, as for example salesmen and research interviewers. Dominance is produced by such factors as age, sex and social class. It can be enhanced by self-presentation, indicating the expertise and experience of the performer, and by assertiveness skills designed to increase the amount of influence over other people. The key to assertion and persuasion is the effective use of verbal requests. They should be made politely, asking rather than ordering, giving reasons which will appeal to the other — 'Come and do the washing up while I change, then we will be able to get to the pub earlier' — and perhaps neutralizing objections — 'There isn't much, you can just put it in the dishwasher'. The verbal request should be accompanied by the appropriate NV manner: an amount of NV dominance which is appropriate to the relationship and conveying a positive attitude to the other. Assertion must be distinguished from aggressiveness, though it may include getting the other to do something he doesn't really want to do — he is offered interpersonal rewards in exchange.

However, there is more to relationships than friendship and dominance. The concepts like those which were used for situations can also be used for relationships.

Goals We have studied the goals and goal structure for nurses and patients, and the results are shown in Figure 1.4. This shows that the only conflict seen by nurses is between the bodily well-being of the nurses and the patients.

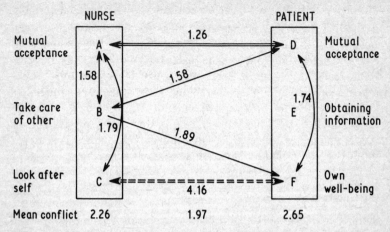

Figure 1.4 The goal structure of nurse–patient encounters (from Graham *et al.*, 1980).

Activities We have studied the activities engaged in by people in a variety of relationships. Friends eat, drink, talk, may engage in joint leisure activities, but do not usually work together. Disliked colleagues at work are seen, if at all, at brief and formal meetings or at morning coffee. Spouses are seen much more than anyone else, and especially have intimate conversations, do domestic jobs together, eat informal meals and argue.

Rules Some of the rules discovered for situations also include relationships, e.g. with doctors and tutors. Work is in hand to find the main rules for the main kind of relationships.

Many skills have special problems in the sphere of relationships. Nurses, for example, have to make and break quite intimate relationships (p. 41), doctors, psychotherapists and others have to maintain a certain 'distance' from their patients. Supervisors have to maintain their position as task leaders and also keep on friendly terms with the group.

Beginning a new relationship may require more than just social skill. Some relationships call for self-confidence or other aspects of self-image, an emotional preparedness to deal with the possibilities and consequences, a sufficient interest in other people and concern for their welfare, as well as relevant technical skills or knowledge.

Self-presentation

The self is a cognitive system which plays an important part in social behaviour. In particular, it is responsible for self-presentation, embarrassment, and phenomena such as stage fright. The *self-image* refers to the way a person perceives himself. It includes roles − like occupation, social class and religion − 'personality' qualities like 'intelligent' or 'kind', and perceptions of the body − e.g. as attractive, tall or fat. The self-image can be assessed by the Twenty Statements Test, which has 20 identical questions ('Who am I?'). Another method is the Semantic Differential; the self is rated on a series of seven-point scales like *warm - - - - - - - cold*. The *ego-ideal* is an important part of the self-system. It can be assessed by asking people to rate 'The kind of person I would most like to be' on seven-point scales. The discrepancies between self and ego-ideal can be readily seen. *Self-esteem* is the extent to which a person accepts and approves of himself. It can be deduced from the average discrepancy between self-image and ego-ideal, but it is better to use self-ratings on evaluation scales like good−bad, nice−nasty. There are also differences in the *degrees of integration* of the self, varying from those who have a completely integrated pattern of life to those who, like children, do not yet know who they are or where they are going.

The origins of self-image and self-esteem are now fairly clear.

The reactions of others

The 'looking glass' theory of the self suggested that we acquire self-images through learning the reactions of others. There is a certain amount of experimental evidence that the judgments of those whose opinions are respected become part of the self-image, though such judgments have less effect after an integrated identity has been established.

Comparisons

These are made with siblings, friends and those in the same form or neighbourhood. Indeed terms like 'tall' or 'clever' are only meaningful in comparison with others.

Roles played

These affect the self-image, as when medical students come to see themselves as doctors. However, people often combine a role and a trait, so a person might see himself as a *scientific* doctor, expressing a degree of 'role-distance'.

Identification with models

This affects the ideal self — a person admires the model and wants to be like him. It also affects the self-image, since he feels that he is already like the model. Identification with the same-sex parent is one of the main origins of feeling and behaving like a male or a female.

Adolescent identity crisis

Erikson (1956) observed that between 16 and 24 young people feel increasing pressures to decide about a career, a marital partner, a political and religious outlook and a lifestyle. Before they acquire an integrated identity they may go through various unsuccessful resolutions, such as conflict between two or more alternative identities, and postponing these decisions, e.g. until after college.

The self is not at work all the time but is activated by particular kinds of situation. Being in front of an audience makes people feel self-conscious and often anxious. There are many situations where people may regard others as audiences. Duval and Wicklund (1972) called this state 'objective self-awareness' — being aware of oneself as an object for others. People are also made self-conscious if they are in some way different from everyone else present, such as being the only female present. Conversely 'de-individuation' can be brought about by dressing everyone up alike. Self-awareness is brought about by penetration of territory or privacy, or unintended self-disclosure. Some people feel more self-conscious than others, and suffer more from audience anxiety. They tend to be people who are shy, have rather low self-esteem and have failed to form an integrated identity.

When the self is activated, there is heightened physiological arousal, and greater concern with the impression made on others. This can be controlled to some extent by 'self-presentation', i.e. sending information about the self. This is done partly to sustain self-esteem, and partly for professional purposes — teachers teach more effectively if their pupils think they are well informed, for example. If people tell others how good they are in words, this is regarded as a joke and disbelieved, at least in western cultures. Jones (1964) found that verbal ingratiation is done with subtlety — e.g. drawing attention to assets in unimportant areas. Most self-presentation is done non-verbally: by clothes, hair style, accent, badges and general style of behaviour. Social class is very clearly signalled in these ways, as is membership of rebellious social groups (Argyle 1975). Self-presentation is needed in all social skills, but especially in those which require performance in front of an audience, like presenting, or where it is important to win the confidence of clients, as in doctor–patient skill.

Physical attractiveness (p.a.) can be regarded as part of self-presentation, since it is partly, even mainly, under an individual's control. Attention to clothes, hair and skin, binding or padding, height of shoes or hat, diet and exercise, facial expression and posture can do a great deal for p.a. People who are attractive are believed, rightly or wrongly, to be superior in all sorts of ways, are liked more, and are treated better (Berscheid and Walster 1964). The faces of mental patients are less attractive than those of controls, partly because they were less attractive before they became patients and partly because they became less attractive while being patients (Napoleon *et al.* 1980).

Goffman (1956) maintained that social behaviour includes a great deal of deceptive self-presentation, by individuals and groups, which is often in the interest of those deceived, as in the work of morticians and doctors. In everyday life, deception is probably less common than concealment. Most people keep quiet about discreditable events in their past, and others don't remind them. Stigmatized individuals like homosexuals, drug addicts and members of certain professions also keep the source of stigma concealed, though they are usually recognized by other members. Goffman's theory gives an explanation of embarrassment — this occurs when false self-presentation is unmasked. Later research has shown that this is the case, but that embarrassment also occurs when other people break social rules and when social accidents are committed — unintentional gaffes, and forgetting names, for example (Argyle 1969).

References

Argyle, M. (1967). *The Psychology of Interpersonal Behaviour*. Harmonds-worth: Penguin (3rd edition 1978).

_____ (1969). *Social Interaction*. London: Methuen.

_____ (1972). *The Social Psychology of Work*. London: Allen Lane, The Penguin Press.

_____ (1975). *Bodily Communication*. London: Methuen.

Argyle, M. (ed.) (1981). *Social Skills and Work*. London: Methuen.

Argyle, M. and Dean, J. (1965). Eye-contact, distance and affiliation. *Sociometry* 28, 289–304.

Argyle, M. and Kendon, A. (1967). The experimental analysis of social performance. *In* Berkowitz, L. (ed.). *Advances in Experimental Social Psychology*. New York: Academic Press, vol. 3, pp. 55–98.

Argyle, M. and Cook, M. (1976). *Gaze and Mutual Gaze*. Cambridge University Press.

Argyle, M., Lefebvre, L. and Cook, M. (1974). The meaning of five patterns of gaze. *Eur. J. Soc. Psychol.* 4, 385–402.

Argyle, M., Furnham, A. and Graham, J. A. (1981). *Social Situations*. Cambridge University Press.

Argyle, M., Graham, J. A., Campbell, A. and White, P. (1979). The rules of different situations. *N. Z. Psychologist* 8, 13–22.

Argyle, M., Salter, V., Nicholson, H., Williams, M. and Burgess, P. (1970). The communication of inferior and superior attitudes by verbal and non-verbal signals. *Br. J. Soc. Clin. Psychol.* 9, 221–31.

Bales, R. F. (1950). *Interaction Process Analysis*. Cambridge, Mass.: Addison-Wesley.

Beattie, G. W. (1980). The skilled art of conversational interaction: verbal and non-verbal signals in its regulation and management. *In* Singleton, W. T., Spurgeon, P. and Stammers, R. B. (eds). *The Analysis of Social Skill*. New York and London: Plenum, pp. 193–211.

Berscheid, E. and Walster, E. (1964). Physical Attractiveness. *In* Berkowitz, L. (ed.). *Advances in Experimental Social Psychology*. New York: Academic Press, vol. 1, pp. 158–215.

Buck, R. (1979). Individual differences in nonverbal sending accuracy and electrodermal responding: the extermalizing-internalizing dimension. *In* Rosenthal, R. (ed.). *Skill in Non-verbal Communication*. Cambridge, Mass.: Oelgeschlager, Gunn and Hain.

Davitz, J. R. (1964). *The Communication of Emotional Meaning*. New York: McGraw-Hill.

Duck, S. (ed.). (1977). *Theory and Practice in Interpersonal Attraction*. London: Academic Press.

Duncan, S. and Fiske, D. W. (1977). *Face-to-Face Interaction: Research Methods and Theory*. New Jersey: Erlbaum.

Ekman, P., Friesen, W. V. and Ellsworth, P. (1972). *Emotion in the Human Face*. Elmsford, N.Y.: Pergamon.

Endler, N. S. and Magnusson, D. (eds) (1976). *Interactional Psychology and Personality*. Washington: Hemisphere.

Flanders, N. A. (1970). *Analyzing Teaching Behavior*. Reading, Mass.: Addison-Wesley.

Flavel, J. H. (1968). *The Development of Role-taking and Communication Skills in Children*. New York: Wiley.

Giles, H. and Powesland, P. F. (1975). *Speech Style and Social Evaluation*. London: Academic Press.

Goffman, E. (1956). *The Presentation of Self in Everyday Life*. Edinburgh University Press.

Goffman, E. (1971). *Relations in Public: Microstudies of the Public Order*. Harmondsworth: Penguin Books.

Graham, J. A., Argyle, M. and Furnham, A. (1980). The goal structure of situations. *Eur. J. Soc. Psychol.* 10, 345–66.

Harré, R. and Secord, P. (1972). *The Explanation of Social Behaviour*. Oxford: Blackwell.

Hochschild, A. R. (1979). Emotion, work, feeling rules and social structure. *Am. J. Sociol.* 85, 551–75.

Jones, E. E. (1964). *Ingratiation: a Social Psychological Analysis*. New York: Appleton-Century-Crofts.

Jones, E. E. and Nisbett, R. E. (1972). The actor and the observer: divergent perception of the causes of behavior. *In* Jones, E. E. *et al.* (eds). *Attribution: Perceiving the Causes of Behavior*. Morristown, N.J.: General Learning Press.

Kendon, A. (1967). Some functions of gaze direction in social interaction. *Acta Psychol.* 26, 22–63.

Mehrabian, A. (1971). *Nonverbal Communication*. Chicago: Aldine-Atherton.

Mischel, W. (1968). *Personality and Assessment*. New York: Wiley.

Napoleon, T., Chassin, L. and Young, R. D. (1980). A replication and extension of 'Physical attractiveness and mental illness'. *J. Abnorm. Psychol.* 89, 250–53.

Patterson, M. (1973). Compensation in non-verbal immediacy behaviors: a review. *Sociometry* 36, 237–352.

Patterson, M. (1976). An arousal model of interpersonal intimacy. *Psychol. Rev.* 83, 235–45.

Romano, J. M., and Bellack, A. S. (1980). Social validation of a component model of assertive behavior. *J. Consult. Clin. Psychol.* 48, 478–90.

Rommetveit, R. (1974). *On Message Structure*. London: Wiley.

Rosenfeld, H. M. (1978). Conversational control functions of nonverbal behaviour. *In* Siegman, A. W. and Feldstein, S. (eds). *Nonverbal Behavior and Communication*. Hillsdale, N.J.: Erlbaum.

Tagiuri, R. (1958). Social preference and its perception. *In* Tagiuri, R. and Petrullo, L. (eds). *Person Perception and Interpersonal Behavior*. Stanford: Stanford University Press.

Trower, P. (1980). Situational analysis of the components and processes of socially skilled and unskilled patients. *J. Consult. Clin. Psychol.* 48, 327–39.

Wish, M. and Kaplan, S. J. (1977). Toward an implicit theory of interpersonal communication. *Sociometry* 40, 234–46.

2 Social skills in nursing

BRYN DAVIS

Introduction

Nursing is called a caring profession. Not only is the nurse expected to care for physical needs of patients, but also for socio-economic needs. Calling nursing a profession implies that there is a system to the caring that is practised, drawing on a body of knowledge and requiring training in that practice. However, nursing often seems to consist of routines applied without 'rhyme or reason' (Chapman 1976), based on tradition and tending to concentrate on physical skills and care.

This concentration on physical skills and care perhaps reflects the enormous developments in technical aspects of treatment with which the nurse has become involved over the last 50 years or so. In the last century, when care was less sophisticated, there was greater weight to Florence Nightingale's advice to nurses that the patient 'feels what a convenience it would be if there were any single person to whom he could speak simply and openly'. She also argued that although this was a means of giving pleasure to the sick, the nurse should be warned against 'absurd consolations . . . absurd statistical comparisons made common conversation by the most sensible people for the benefit of the sick' and against 'pulling the string . . . of this showerbath of silly hopes and encouragements'. Miss Nightingale told nurses that 'they like you to be fresh, lively and interested' (1970, p. 55).

Concern with the quality of care implies the establishment of ways of making assessments. Great interest has been expressed in the question of nursing outcomes. Kelman (1976) argues that they must be operationalized, observable, measurable, relevant and valid criteria, related to nursing activities. This assumes that there are outcomes that are primarily attributable to nursing care, and that these can be identified. With reference to communication and social skills, Bloch (1975) refers to psychosocial, cognitive and behavioural aspects of health status, but sees them as intermediate outcomes, implying that they are not legitimate outcomes in themselves. Outcomes can surely be in terms of psychosocial, cognitive and behavioural criteria if these are assessed as the patient's needs.

The question of assessment and outcome is taken up later, and is of great importance to the subject of social skills in nursing. However preliminary discussion of other aspects of social skills must be undertaken before we can consider them. The first part of this chapter concerns the need for social skills in nursing, and involves the profession, the patients and the clinical need. This part is followed by a discussion of problems in nurse–patient relationships; nurses talking to patients, and the influence of organizational and personality factors. Finally, a solution is offered, involving the assessment of and training in social skills.

The need for social skills in nursing

The profession

The quotations from Florence Nightingale's *Notes for Nurses* show that she recognized the importance to patients of nurses practising social skills, being interested in patients, and not giving them routine, impersonal or 'absurd' consolations but being prepared to lend an ear. Very few modern nursing textbooks give as much importance to this aspect of nursing. Two notable exceptions, one British the other American, are Roper (1973) and Henderson and Nite (1978).

The General Nursing Councils of England and Wales and of Scotland are responsible for the education and accreditation of nurses and for the maintenance of a Register of Nurses. The syllabus laid down by the GNC for England and Wales lists, among many other topics, the relationship between the nurse, patients and relatives, the place of the nurse in the hospital team, relationships with medical staff and other health workers. There is also a special section of subjects under human behaviour in relation to illness, including the effects of coming into hospital, the nurse–patient relationship and relation between emotional states and physical conditions. Under the section Study of Man and his Environment the syllabus includes personal and impersonal behaviour in groups (GNC 1977). In the new modular scheme of training which the GNC for Scotland has recently published, the role of the nurse for each module is itemized, including nurse–patient relationships relative to the emphasis of the module, perception of the patient's needs as a person, conversation, information and education needs (GNC 1978).

A random sample of nurses from four hospital groups in Scotland were asked if they were generally able to give enough time to patients or if they would like to be able to give more time to them. They were also asked, if they would like to give more time to patients, how they would utilize the time. Of the 588 respondents, two-thirds indicated they would like more time. The most common uses to which extra time would be put included communication, talking and listening, reassurance and explanation (Hockey 1976).

The patients

Many attempts to study the patients' attitudes to hospitals, to nursing care or to communication have been undertaken over the last few decades. All have produced similar results. For example, a survey of twelve randomly selected districts in England and Wales, involving 739 people who had been in hospital in the previous six months, showed that 60 per cent reported difficulty in getting the information they required about their illness, treatment, progress and tests (Cartwright 1964). They were more critical of this aspect than anything else. A relationship was found between 'need to know' and 'dissatisfaction'. 70 per cent reported that they received no information from nurses. 11 per cent said that the nurse was the main source of information. However, in the interviews many comments were made explaining these responses, saying that information was not the nurses' job, or that nurses cannot speak out of turn. 44 per cent felt that Sister gave no information; 40 per cent that she gave a little; 16 per cent that she gave a lot. There was also a tendency that if the patient was not given information by the Sister then the doctor was also not found helpful. Patients expressed difficulty in knowing whom to ask.

This report of criticism of communication is supported by other studies since then, for example by McGee (1961) and Levitt (1975), both of them small-scale single-hospital studies. Support also comes from Franklin (1974), in a study of four male surgical wards in four different hospitals, from Carstairs (1970) in a survey of most of the hospitals in Scotland — where nurses' attitudes were appreciated but the social environment and information caused dissatisfaction — and from Raphael who surveyed both general and psychiatric hospitals (1977*a*, *b*). The Royal Commission on the Health Service reported dissatisfaction with information-giving about progress, from both in- and outpatients (HMSO 1978). A study of relationships in a day hospital reported that the patients valued their relationships with nurses most highly, with social workers least highly and with doctors in an intermediate position (Ferguson and Carney 1970).

This need is typically associated with nurses. Thus we have the leaders of the profession claiming a role for nurses including communications and human relations, and at the same time there is in patients a need for communication and in particular for information. The simple answer seems to be that nurses should spend more time in communication with patients. Unfortunately, it seems that not all the patients wish for information; rather, all patients would like a certain amount of information, for the evidence referred to above indicates that some patients were satisfied with the R communications they received. Evidence from recent unpublished surveys indicates that some patients would not like to know too much, and prefer that nurses should not interact indiscriminately. Discretion is called for on the part of the nurses, a point that will be taken up later on.

The clinical need

We have seen evidence of a professional need to communicate, to be involved in human relations, and a felt need by patients for the exercise of these skills, with particular reference to information giving. Is there a clinical need for the nurse to engage in communication; to use her social skills? Is there any evidence of patient outcomes being influenced by these factors?

The main evidence of an effect of interpersonal relations on patient outcomes has been from studies of preoperative information giving and postoperative outcomes. The rationale is usually that of stress from anxiety being reduced in association with the information giving, resulting in psychological and physiological changes and improvements in postoperative progress.

Two studies in the UK have reviewed the literature in this field and have themselves disclosed significant changes. Hayward (1975) used a psychological measure of anxiety, the S—R Inventory, which he correlated with the Eysenck Personality Inventory (EPI). He showed a reduction in anxiety, and also found significant differences between experimental and control patients for analgesic consumption. Informed patients received significantly fewer drugs and also, using a 'pain thermometer', became relatively pain-free more rapidly than the controls. They reported better sleep and a quicker return to normal appetite. Hayward acknowledges, however, the difficulties in measuring these variables.

Boore's (1978) study used physiological measure of stress for the main variable (the presence of 17-hydroxycorticosteroids and the sodium:potassium ratio in the urine). There was some evidence for lower 17-hydroxycorticosteroid excretion in the informed group but not for a difference in sodium:potassium ratios. The informed group also had significantly fewer postoperative wound infections. There were no significant differences regarding analgesic consumption, pain, morale or physical state. A high negative correlation was demonstrated between physical state and 17-hydroxycorticosteroid excretion, physical state being measured by the Recovery Inventory devised by Wolfer and Davis (1970). This assesses patients' perceptions of sleep, appetite, strength, stomach condition, bowel condition, urination, self-assistance and movement.

The effects of information on stress associated with hospital investigations has been demonstrated by Wilson-Barnett (1979), who also related the stress reactions to personality traits, using the Mood Adjective Check List and the EPI.

The question of communications as a hospital factor has been related to patient outcomes by Revans (1964). He reported an increase in length of patient stay being associated with the internal hospital communications, assessed as Sisters' opinions of senior staff and Sisters' attitudes to student nurses, and in particular found a higher correlation with length of patient stay for medical patients than for surgical patients. This, he suggested, was due to the greater dependence of medical patients on social skills for diagnosis and treatment.

Therapeutic effects have been noted in the psychiatric setting too. Gruen studied eighty-five 'privileged long-stay patients' (1970). He found conflicting aims between departments and a lack of communication about these to the patients by the staff. Patients did not know the name or purpose of the drugs they were being given, the purpose of the rehabilitation programme, or the criteria by which the nurses assessed them for recommendations for discharge. Gruen argued that poor communications help to increase the long-term nature of the patient's illness. Another study, of small group interactions in a thirty-five-bed male ward for long-stay patients, showed an effect on personal habits, general behaviour, interpersonal relationships and work performance. These were, however, rated by the nurses, who were also the leaders in the groups: a serious methodological weakness. Altschul (1972) in a study in one psychiatric hospital found that a small number of patients saw their interactions with nurses as therapeutic. This study is discussed in more detail in the next section.

Thus both positive and negative outcomes have been highlighted, although much more work needs to be done to show their full dynamics and control. Some of the studies quoted do suffer from methodological weaknesses, for example, which reduce the effect of their findings. Both Hayward and Boore manipulated what can be seen as two separate variables − that is, information giving and patients' coping strategies. Johnston, *et al.* (1978) have discussed this and offer findings from an experiment that show that both these variables have individual and combined effects, and are related to nurse−patient interactions which use nurses' social skills.

The problem of nurse−patient relationships

Nurses talking to patients

Although nursing is seen as using human relations and communication skills, although patients have repeatedly been shown to need these and to comment on their inadequacy, and although there is a developing body of evidence relating these skills to patients' clinical outcomes, nurses themselves do not seem to place much importance in practising these skills. One important study found that nurse−patient interaction, when it occurred, was task related (Stockwell 1972). Thirty-six nurses when interviewed did not consider conversations with patients as 'work' and felt guilty about them. The nurses also tended not to be available to patients if there were no tasks to be done, and quite often many tasks were carried out without words between nurse and patient. The patients felt that the nurses were too busy to be bothered with trivial matters. Observations supplementary to the interviews showed that nurses were selective in their conversations with patients. The more popular patients were those who were able to communicate readily, who knew the nurse's name and who co-operated in their treatment. The nurses spent more time with these patients, whom they regarded as individuals, allowed to give gifts and undertook favours for, and for whom they allowed lapses in the rules.

In this study it was also shown that nurses used sanctions against patients who complained or grumbled, who expressed lack of enjoyment, or who expressed more suffering than was believed to be warranted by the nurses. These patients were ignored, had their gifts or favours refused, had rules rigidly enforced and were treated with sarcasm. These results suggest that nurses have certain role expectations for patients. Further evidence of nurses' expectations of patients was provided by Johnston (1976) who studied the relationships between forty-eight patients and nineteen nurses in three gynaecological wards over the immediate postoperative period. The Hospital Adjustment Inventory (HAI) of de Wolfe, *et al.* (1966) was used, measuring psychological distress, together with the Recovery Inventory of Wolfer and Davis (1970), measuring physical feelings. These inventories were given to patients and nurses in an attempt to correlate the predictions of nurses with the experiences of the patients. The findings indicated that nurses underestimated the patients' physical distress but overestimated their worries. There was little significant correlation between individual pairs of nurse and patient with the HAI as to which individual patients had which worries (only thirteen pairs were significantly positively correlated out of forty-eight pairs). However, nurses did predict generally which worries most patients would have. Similarly, with perception of patients' physical state, there was a tendency for the nurses' predictions to be better at the general level than at the particular, individual level.

These two studies suggest that nurses have stereotyped perceptions of patients and interact with them accordingly. That is, they deal with the typical or average patient, not with the individual. A patient who breaks the stereotype − who is not appreciative, sociable, or offers different physical or psychological symptoms from those expected − will tend to be ignored, forgotten or treated with sarcasm.

In the specific instance of dying patients, it seems that nurses (district nurses and health visitors in particular) feel that it is their responsibility to give hope and support, not information (see Nightingale 1970). This view is supported by doctors, who prefer nurses to inspire hope and a positive outcome, or to refer questions about prognosis to the doctor − if possible the patient's own doctor − or to do both of these (Cartwright, Hockey and Anderson 1973).

Despite this rather negative evidence about nurses' attitudes and practices with regard to nurse−patient communication, nurses do claim that talking with patients is an important nursing role. Anderson (1973) looked at the patients and staff in three hospitals: small, medium and large. This included 156 patients, 79 nurses and 75 doctors. She asked these three groups to rank ten roles of the nurse in order of importance. Nurses ranked 'talking with patients' second, doctors ranked it third and patients ranked it fourth. In support of the importance of nurses and their role as communicators, 66 per cent of patients reported that they were upset by emotional aspects of their stay, giving as examples: boredom, discourteous staff and communication problems. Many related their emotional upset to their own personal fears, loneliness and confusion. 93 per cent of nurses' responses referred to patients having emotional upsets. This supports the findings of Johnston (1976) that nurses are aware of the upsets to which patients are usually susceptible.

The problem seems to be that nurses do not know how to talk to patients as individuals, what to say or how to say it. Observational studies have attempted to analyse nurse−patient conversations. Kerrigan (1957), in the USA, observed thirty-two student nurses during their first clinical experience, and analysed their conversations with patients according to categories of responding. These included passivity, responsiveness, development, divergence, change of topic or negative response. Of the students' responses, 50 per cent were inadequate or ignored the point. 72 per cent of the students' responses to patients' initial questions about themselves or their family were negative, leading to the termination of the conversation. The students seemed to work mainly in category 1, passive but attentive, with only 35 per cent of items being responding and developing (categories 2 and 3). Much use was made of category 4, change of topic.

This study concerned students at an early stage of training when one might expect inadequate and unskilled behaviour. The type of training is also very different to that practised in the UK, where a study of patterns of ward management including a study of nurse−patient conversations − of experienced nurses and learners − was carried out by Moult, Melia and Pembrey (1978). All patients on four wards in three hospitals were observed for a total of 6.75 hours, note being taken on an activity-coding sheet of all activities performed by nurses with or for them. One of the hypotheses was that nurses talk with patients only when performing some physical aspect of their care. This was supported by the findings. The average length of conversation not linked with other activity was forty-five seconds. Conversations were commonly begun by nurses and terminated by them, even when begun by patients. Conversation in this study was defined as 'any verbal exchange between nurse and patient, however brief or superficial' (ibid., p. 115).

Another British study attempted to analyse nurse–patient conversations using radio microphones and tape-recording equipment (Faulkner 1979). The microphones were worn by the nurses for one and a half hours during the morning and evening periods. The recordings were analysed under three categories – social, task and disease – and each category was further coded into fifteen types of interaction. Again most conversation was found to be task orientated, and least was found to be disease orientated. Nurses avoided answering questions about the disease or treatment. In this study, the data were 'pieces of conversation', i.e. uninterrupted speech from one individual.

Both Kerrigan and Faulkner showed nurses' inadequacy in conversation, their reluctance to enter into lengthy discussions, their tendency to change the topic, and otherwise avoid questions. Faulkner and Moult *et al.* also indicated the control that the nurse has over the conversations and in particular over their termination.

In psychiatry one would assume that talking with patients would be regarded as work and would be undertaken more readily, be longer and more relevant to the patients' needs. In a study in one psychiatric hospital forty nurses' interactions with 115 patients were observed (Altschul 1972). The number of interactions and their length were recorded. The nurses' reports of the interactions were assessed and the patients and nurses were interviewed about the interactions. Most interactions were concerned with social conversations or physical care (42.6 and 35.1 per cent respectively), the remainder being concerned with psychological problems (25.1 per cent). However, when analysed by length of time, most was spent on psychological problems (38.5 per cent) with slightly less on aspects of physical care and social conversation (37.3 and 34.8 per cent respectively). The interactions were also influenced by diagnosis, with a large proportion of patients not interacting at all (40 per cent). Some diagnostic groups accounted for a major part of the interactions, in particular organic mental disorders and the physically ill. Depressed or neurotic patients had the least interactions. When interviewed, however, nurses admitted to no rationale behind their interactions, claiming chance or intuition. There was a significant correlation between rate of interaction and being seen as helpful by the patient. This echoes the finding by Stockwell (1972).

Altschul also found a significant correlation between interaction rate and being known by name by the patient. Twelve patient–nurse pairs were found where there was reciprocity as to the reports of a special relationship, eleven of these patients finding the relationship therapeutic. The nurses in the pairs were observed to have a longer average interaction time and a higher rate of interaction, as also did the patients, which suggests an association between the rate and time of interactions and their being seen as therapeutic, although this group was too small for statistical confirmation.

In another single-hospital study the work of three charge nurses was observed in a long-stay unit containing twenty female patients and thirty-nine male patients (Cheadle 1971). Interaction times were again related to diagnosis or symptoms and also length of patient stay. The shortest interactions were associated with withdrawn or incoherent patients. Yet another study of charge nurses in psychiatric hospitals observed their interactions with patients, and again diagnosis influenced the interactions, with schizophrenic patients and psychopaths receiving more than expected. There were less interactions than expected with depressed and neurotic patients as well as with those suffering from hypomania and paranoia.

Hence, nurses seem to be selective in their interactions with patients. This could be influenced by the type of feedback they receive. This conclusion seems to apply both to the general and psychiatric fields. The choice is rarely reported to have a therapeutic rationale, most interactions being associated with tasks performed for the patients, or occurring as a result of chance or intuition. The interactions, particularly in the general field, can be of very short duration; only with certain groups of psychiatric patients do they attain any reasonable length.

The influence of organizational factors

Nurses do not work in isolation, but are part of a complex organization of sub-systems making up the profession. This has a definite hierarchical structure, and within that structure there is a constant interplay between individual personality factors and organizational influences.

Using a psychodynamic approach and insights gained from studies of relations in industry, Menzies (1960) studied the nursing social system in a general hospital, where there were problems relating to the allocation of students to the wards. High levels of stress, tension and anxiety were found, and defensive techniques operating within the social system of the nursing service were identified. The system requires intimacy between nurses and patients, and yet expects the nurses to move frequently from ward to ward, breaking off developing relationships. The defensive measures operating to reduce this strain tend to produce secondary anxieties, without adequately solving the primary anxiety. An important concept, taken from industry, is that of discretion, the responsibility for certain levels of decision making. In nursing Menzies found a persistent elimination of this aspect of responsibility, and refers to the conflict caused by the removal of this means of obtaining personal satisfaction.

The study just described deals with subjective interpretive material rather than empirical data. Later studies have attempted to be more objective. Another report, for example, has similarly described the hospital as an organism characterized by anxiety (Revans 1972) and functioning as a cycle of anxiety, uncertainty and communication blockage. In the report this is related to 'a will to communicate' which is part of the 'concept of organism' (ibid., pp. 93–94). Revans found that the Sisters' attitudes to status and seniority, to the integration of the students with their training, and to the organization were a significant hospital characteristic. It was shown that the students' relations with the Sister were directly related to Sisters' own relations with her senior. Revans suggested that this relationship between the students and Sister may influence the students' relationships with the patient.

The possibility of a therapeutic influence is supported by some evidence from the USA. Cassee (1975) reports a study of intra-professional relations and nurse–patient relations. He found a positive correlation between the incidence of therapeutic behaviour and openness between nurses. From the results of a factor analysis of the data it was shown that nurse–patient socioemotional communication occurred only when nurse–nurse communication was emotionally, open. This latter type of communication was defined as free discussion of the way the unit was functioning, allowing consultation between nurses about particular patient care and encouraging discussion about differences. The emotionally open, nurse—patient relationship was described as supporting the patient with his problems and difficulties, talking about his anxieties concerning his illness and asking his opinion about treatments. Leonard (1975) has studied the nature and effects of hospital climate based on staff interpersonal relationships and therapeutic ideology. The aim was to assess the effects of three different ward administration phases in a psychiatric hospital. This was a natural experiment, in that Leonard took advantage of changes occurring as part of the therapeutic development and administrative reorganization in one hospital. An Affect Expression Checklist was used. In terms of nine of the eleven items the last phase was seen negatively, most of these items concerning communications, and Leonard argues that these results provide support for those of Moos and Houts (1970) among others, that patients' perceptions of ward climate correlate highly with their satisfaction with their ability to initiate communication with staff and in group discussions.

The influence of nurses' personality factors

We thus have two strands of evidence coming together from the last two sections: the difficulties that nurses have in communicating and their avoidance of interactions, and the dynamics within the structure of the social system of nursing which can have an influence on the development or use of social skills and relationships. Some hints within these two strands suggest that it is the nurse's own personality traits and reactions to the stresses of the caring role that are a large part of the problem. This point is illustrated by the survey undertaken by Davitz and Davitz (1975) into nurses' reactions to the suffering of patients. On entering clinical experience there seems to be an increased selectivity of reactions leading both to an increase in compassion and yet a more realistic perception. Nurses soon began to assess the 'legitimacy' or otherwise of a patient's complaint of pain and unhappiness, and if this was thought to be unwarranted this led to avoidance or an angry response. Davitz and Davitz also reported the association of guilt with this reaction.

The study also showed that patients who expressed emotional problems of a non-psychiatric nature received little sympathy, and this was explained by the nurses as being due to feelings of helplessness and inadequacy. A common reaction to patients who were seriously ill was one of over-involvement, expressed by the development of empathic symptoms, taking problems home with them, developing an emotional distance or a macabre sense of humour. When dealing with patients who were dying or when patients had died, nurses felt helplessness, anger and despair, and tended to reflect on their own life.

Reactions to progression from school to ward are described by Kramer (1974), who labels them 'reality shock'. Reality is defined as the work experience perceived and shared by groups of nurses. Shock is defined as the total social, physical and emotional response of the person to the unexpected, unwanted or even intolerable. The progression process is described as a pattern of several phases: honeymoon, shock or rejection, recovery and resolution. Coping mechanisms include rejection, protective isolationism, hostile or aggressive attitudes to the host culture, moral outrage, vocal criticism and excessive fatigue. Important aspects of reality shock are the different expectations of the neophyte in the new culture, particularly expectations of competence. These expectations increase the pressure on the newcomer. The training in the USA is full-time college based, and the reality shock refers to the change from college ideals to the ward realities.

Some researchers have looked specifically at nurses' personality traits. One is Cordiner (1968) who used Cattell's 16 PF Questionnaire Form C (IPAT). The scores indicated above-average self-control, conservatism, shyness and soberness. They also indicated below-average self-assurance, forthrightness, emotional maturity and self-discipline. Singh used the same questionnaire (1971) and found general students undergoing the traditional three-year apprenticeship training more cold, aloof, self-contained and shy than students on experimental training schemes. Using the California Test of Personality, the Kuder Preference Record and the Rotter incomplete Sentences Blank, Birch (1975) found that the group as a whole was not adjusted. In particular there was less self-reliance, freedom from nervous symptoms and total personal adjustment on the California Test.

Therefore, there is evidence that nurses are selective in their interactions in relation to the feedback that they might obtain. Interactions are usually task orientated, or occur as a result of chance, and are usually of short duration. There also seem to be aspects of the organization of nursing and nurse–nurse relationships which influence nurse–patient relationships. These two strands are linked by findings that nurses are psychologically vulnerable people in general, possessing characteristics such as low self-assurance, low emotional maturity, lack of self-discipline, high conscientiousness and sensitivity and having trusting natures. The final section deals with attempts which have been made to improve nurses' social skills and suggests directions for further research and development.

A solution: the assessment of and training in social skills

It is becoming increasingly apparent that nurse–patient relationships are complex phenomena, dependent as they are on varying degrees of patient need or desire to know or to communicate, together with varying feelings of anxiety and inadequacy, and varying pressures of conformity to hospital or nursing climates on the part of nurses. This complexity is such that nurses require quite sophisticated skills and training in those skills.

Some authorities naïvely call for more or better communications, assuming that such skills are common sense, inborn not learnt, and only a matter of conscientious application. Others, mainly in the USA, are aware of the complex nature of the situation and attempts have been made both to study ways of training nurses in those skills and, as a necessary adjunct, to study ways of assessing competence in and need for those skills.

Assessment of communications skills

One of the earliest attempts to describe effective and ineffective inter-acting behaviours was that of Hays and Larson (1963). They listed twenty-five therapeutic techniques, illustrating them from clinical material, and nineteen non-therapeutic techniques, illustrating them similarly. These examples were collated from or based on the work of many professionals and teachers concerned with interpersonal relationships in nursing, and were mainly of a psychodynamic nature. The techniques were related largely to psychiatric settings, but many of the non-therapeutic techniques were echoed in the studies of the general field of nursing discussed in the previous sections. Hays and Larson also published the Bachand Problematic Verbal Patterns Tool for analysing student nurses' interactions. Six types of response were assessed, disclosing those that are problematic for the student. No details are given of the validity or reliability of the Tool, which was first described in an unpublished thesis (Bachand 1959).

Since then assessment has been recognized as an important part of social skills training. Hatton (1977) has produced a list of behaviours similar to that of Hays and Larson, but she relates these to the patient's psychosocial needs, suggesting that the list could become a valuable worker-evaluation tool. A Challenge Examination in interpersonal skills is described by Eggert (1975). The technique used is that of videotaped recordings of the students while counselling. One of the most sophisticated studies of the assessment of nurses' interpersonal skills is that of Ryden (1977). This experiment attempted to predict nurses' clinical practice on the basis of social skills assessments. The predictive measures used were a paper-and-pencil test and ratings of simulated interviews after a course on interpersonal skills. The top scorers and the bottom scorers were compared over two years of clinical practice and assessment, the top scorers performing significantly better than the bottom scorers after two years. There was also a significant correlation between the post-course scores and the clinical practice scores. This seems to suggest a predictive value to the post-course assessment. There were no pre-course scores so that the effect of the course itself was not assessed. The rating scales were also highly subjective. There was no clear indication that the raters were ignorant of the post-course scores, and so not biased by them. Nevertheless, this study is a major step forward in the attempt to understand and measure social skills in nursing.

Training in social skills

There is little evidence in the British literature of attempts to implement and evaluate training for nurses in social skills. From the evidence discussed in the earlier sections of this chapter it would seem that there are many aspects to the problem. Sheahan (1976), in one of a series of articles discussing communication in education, identifies eight aspects. These include information giving, kindness, compassion, courtesy and goodwill. However, to plan a training module or to prepare an assessment schedule there should be not only an awareness of the complexity but also an understanding of the problems. The problems identified in the discussion in the previous sections are:

(1) Self-confidence in the nurses, with particular respect to social situations including potential trauma to nurse or patient.
(2) The prevention of defensive behaviours and attitudes in nurses.
(3) The perception and assessment of patients' socioemotional and information needs by nurses.
(4) The development of skills in interactions about socioemotional needs.
(5) Decisions about the discretion available to nurses on the socio-emotional and information needs of patients.
(6) The organization of the nursing service so that patterns of nursing behaviour that are defensive or disrupt nurse—patient relation-ships are avoided.

Items 1—4 in this list include both verbal and non-verbal aspects of communication. NV aspects have not been emphasized in this chapter because there is little in the literature apart from studies of touching (de Wever 1977) and the influences of staff clothing styles (Rinn 1976, Malcolmson, Brandman and Alpert 1977). Many of the studies quoted above, particularly those on problems of nurse—patient relationships, refer to NV reponses of nurses and to NV aspects of patients' behaviour.

If nurses are to develop social skills an integral part of the process is their own personal growth, confidence and freedom from defensive behaviours (items 1 and 2). No British studies have looked at this, although recommendations have been made (Stewart 1975). An American study has been reported (La Monica, *et al.* 1976); this study, and also that of Ceriale (1976), is based on the work and methods of Carkhuff (1969) and Jourard (1971), among others. La Monica and her co-workers describe an experiment to study the effect of a human relations staff development programme. The dependent variable was the Carkhuff Index of Communication (1969), which is claimed to offer an objective measure of level of empathy. Although significant differences were found between the experimental group experiencing the new programme and the control groups, the study did not include the transfer of these effects to practical settings, nor long-term effects, even though Carkhuff does claim such transfer. Ceriale describes the introduction of similar sessions but uses sub-jective reports from the students for evaluation (1976). However, she does show the need for an objective tool, and argues for a long-term study and for clinical transfer.

Assertiveness training, as used in psychiatry, is now being extended to health service staff and to nurses in particular. Few studies of this have been published. In the USA Manderino (1977) reported the findings of an experiment designed to assess the effect of group assertive training and also to relate these to locus of control. Using the Lawrence Assertive Inventory and the Behavioral Assertiveness Test, highly significant differences due to training were found between matched pairs of undergraduate women. No relationship was found between locus of control and the other measures. No attempt was made to assess long-term effects or to validate the findings in practice. A similar exercise was reported by Turner (1976) and by Huber and Hansen (1975).

One study has included an experimental assessment of the effects of a personal growth programme (Farrell 1977). This used videotaped vignettes and standardized instruments designed by Carkhuff (1969) as the dependent variables, followed by peer group and instructor ratings of videotaped recordings of interviews. Again, although significant differences were obtained on post-test measures, no attempt was made to evaluate long-term effects in the clinical setting.

Few of these studies have attempted to relate the programmes to the nurses' emotional or personality or communications needs. Pre-tests were used only for comparison with post-tests. Stewart (1975), while recommending such programmes, also recommends a one-to-one relationship between trainer and trainee, moving slowly from the known (tasks) to the unknown (feelings). Smith (1977) reports the establishment of a workshop plan for the staff of a health centre, consisting of two 4-hour sessions one week apart. The activities were concerned with stumbling blocks to communication that had been identified by the director. These included language, perceptual differences, anxiety and prejudices. Unfortunately, the weakness of the exercise is, again, poor evaluation of the effects. Subjective reports indicated increased satisfaction and commitment to the practice, and a significant utilization of the techniques in interdepartmental communications. Smith suggests that further follow-up sessions would be beneficial and that instructors should be involved in evaluation to offer feedback. One stumbling block to communication not dealt with in the workshop is that of high anxiety. Nevertheless, this study does try to relate content of programme to identified blocks, however general these may be.

Chapman (1976) agrees that as well as patient needs it is also necessary to be concerned with nurses' needs, including needs for empathy and communication skills. She recommends that situations analysis can be used to develop these. Such analysis can include the use of videotapes, role play and case-history material. Miltz (1977) recommends microteaching for the improvement of personal communication. This breaks down the skill into its component parts. It is based on a teach–reteach service offering feedback, including videotape feedback. Miltz reported positive subjective nurses' comments, but as with the studies discussed above did not attempt to evaluate these clinically. Carpenter and Kroth (1976) used a ten-item Behavior Questionnaire in a matched pairs design, with a post-test control group. The aim of the study was to compare the effects of microteaching exercises with non-directive group processes, using a control group studying pharmacology. Although significant results were reported, indicating stronger effects with the microteaching method, the evaluation was done by means of a Self Rating Tool, and consequently there are reservations as to the value to be placed on these findings. Clinical validation with a third person or some more objective rating is essential for full evaluation of these training techniques.

A British study attempting to co-ordinate these methods in an experimental evaluation design has shown some significant results (Davis 1981; Davis and Ternulf-Nyhlin 1981). Pre- and post-course assessments of attitudes and intentions regarding communications and relationships in the hospital setting, and of videotaped interviews with a role-played patient, were obtained from an experimental and a control group of trained staff in a surgical unit. The course involved microteaching of interviewing skills, non-verbal exercises, role play with videotaped feed back and discussions. Significant changes in the directions predicted were found for attitudes and intentions of those nurses selected for the course. Patient and nurse teacher evaluations of the videotaped interviews also found significant or almost significant improvements in the predicted directions for the experimental group.

In the psychiatric field, Smith (1979) has described but not evaluated a method of interaction recordings with nurses.

Referring back to the list of six problem areas identified from the literature, items (3), (5) and (6) do not seem to have been tackled in any great depth yet, although item (3), the perception and assessment of patients' socioemotional and information needs by nurses, is to a certain extent included in the studies just described. Nevertheless, specific attempts to develop such skills and procedures are required and this is being recognized on both sides of the Atlantic, with the development of patient-care plans and patient profiles to prepare such plans. Mackie, Alexander and Grubb (1979) have described the efforts within one hospital to introduce these procedures. The patient profile is a questionnaire from which it is possible to create a picture of the patient's individual needs by enquiring into his activities of daily living relevant to his care by the nursing staff. From this the nursing-care plan can be drawn up, implemented and evaluated. There remains much research and development to be undertaken yet into the most effective profile formats for particular caring situations, as well as into valid evaluation procedures which are related to nursing outcomes.

An international research project, the World Health Organisation Medium Term Programme, Nursing and Midwifery in Europe, is attempting to tackle this problem but as in the USA a major problem is in the definition of nursing outcomes, and nursing situations or diagnoses. Another problem which is related to these is that of the discretion available to nurses with respect to social skills. This must include negotiations about the nurse's role with both health professional and patients. However, if nurses do eventually obtain evidence that they have these skills and that they have beneficial effects of value to the patients then role expectations of social skills for nurses should be more easily acceptable. Studies of the different perceptions of doctors, patients and nurses regarding nurses' social skills are being developed, that of Carlson and Vernon (1973) breaking preliminary ground in the USA.

The organization of inter-nurse relations and the organization of the nursing services is to a certain extent the responsibility of the profession, but because nursing cannot be seen in isolation it must also affect other participants in the health services. Some multidisciplinary studies of intra-hospital relations, communications and innovations show some successes but chiefly highlight the problems (Weiland and Leigh 1971, Revans 1972, Towell and Harries 1979). Studies of organization at ward level (Lelean 1974, Moult, Melia and Pembrey 1978) again show the problems and offer some insights into future directions for research.

Conclusion

This chapter has looked at the question of social skills in nursing from three directions; the needs for them, the problems with them, and some solutions that are being offered. Six aspects of the problem area were presented both to demonstrate its complexity and to begin to formulate the solutions. These aspects include the nurse as a person, the patient as a person to be perceived by the nurse, the development of social skills by the nurse and their assessment, the organization of relationships within the nursing services and with other health professionals, and finally the attitudes of the health professionals and the patients to the use of these skills by nurses. Although communications skills are valued by leading nurse writers, by nurses themselves and by patients, the problems of attaining and performing them are only beginning to be recognized and tackled.

The need for social skills, particularly any therapeutic need, requires further analysis and study to show more clearly the communications roles that can be and should be played by nurses: information giving and receiving, whether solicited by the patient or nurse; problem-solving interactions and the development of emotionally supportive relationships, are all roles in which nurses at some time or other are involved. Each of them demands different variations of social skills, and also the ability to move from one role to another during one interaction. The demands of this superordinate skill of handling a complex variation of communication skills seems to be very threatening both to nurses and to doctors who work with them.

There is much uncertainty as to whether this kind of discretionary role is to be allowed or is wanted by nurses. The giving of information under clearly defined conditions may be a need that can be dealt with by nurses, and it may prove possible to assess nurses' training needs, their attainments, and to provide the training in those skills. Similarly, interviewing skills may be assessed and training devised, as may the other communication skills mentioned above; but whether nurses acquire skills for separate communication procedures, or for a more complex role including a facility for perception and a range of social skills to be used in a discretionary way, depends on whether the nurse is seen as a task-oriented functionary or as being involved in patient-centred planning, of care including nursing outcomes.

It is encouraging to note that within the nursing profession these questions are being actively studied. The survey directed by Hockey (1976) has generated further projects in an attempt to clarify some of the issues. One study has been concerned with patients' fears and worries on planned admission to hospital; another is trying to find out whether nurses value communication in nursing. An evaluative study is monitoring the implementation of the findings of preoperative information-giving studies; and an investigation into the assessment of and training in social skills has been completed (Davis 1981).

The analysis of nurses' conversation skills and the assessment of their social skills on the ward are being studied by current holders of Nursing Research Fellowships funded by the Department of Health and Social Security. The Joint Board of Clinical Nursing Studies is holding workshops to discuss the question of improving social skills in trained nurses, and the National Health Service Learning Resources Unit, Sheffield, is producing material to facilitate communications skills.

This is some of the work currently being undertaken which is directly related to social skills in nursing. There has been insufficient space to allow the discussion of work which has been concerned with the organization of the nursing service and the relations between nurses and other health professionals, such as that described by Towell and Harries (1979), Weiland and Leigh (1971), Revans (1972) and Savage and Widdowson (1974). Nevertheless there is ample evidence of much concern about nurses and their social skills. From the research discussed here it can be seen that a caring profession is recognizing this and beginning to frame the questions to try to gain the answers. It is beginning to write in rhyme and with reason.

References

Altschul, A. T. (1972). *Patient Interaction. A Study of Interaction Patterns in Acute Psychiatric Wards*. Edinburgh: Churchill Livingston.

Anderson, E. R. (1973). *The role of the Nurse*. London: Royal College of Nursing.

Birch, J. (1975). *To Nurse or Not to Nurse*. London: Royal College of Nursing.

Bloch, D. (1975). Evaluation of nursing care in terms of process and outcome. *Nurs. Res.* 24 256–63.

Boore, J. (1978). *Prescription for Recovery*. London: Royal College of Nursing.

Carkhuff, R. R. (1969). *Helping and Human Relations; A Primer for Lay and Professional Helpers. Volume 1. Selection and Training*. New York: Holt, Rinehart and Winston.

Carlson, C. E., Vernon, D. T. A. (1973). Measurement of informativeness of hospital staff members. *Nurs. Res.* 22 198–206.

Carpenter, K. F. and Kroth, J. A. (1976). Effects of videotaped role playing on nurses' therapeutic communications skills. *J. Continuing Education Nurs.* 7, 47–53.

Carstairs, V. (1970). *Channels of Communication*. Scottish Home and Health Department, Number 11.

Cartwright, A. (1964). *Human Relations and Hospital Care*. London: Routledge and Kegan Paul.

Cartwright, A., Hockey, L. and Anderson, J. L. (1973). *Life Before Death*. London: Routledge and Kegan Paul.

Cassee, E. (1975). Therapeutic Behaviour, Hospital Culture and Communication. *In* C. Cox and A. Meade (eds). *Sociology of Medical Practice*. London: Collier Macmillan.

Ceriale, K. (1976). Facilitated unfolding of human relations skills in the baccalaureate nursing student. *Nurse Educator* 1, 11−13.

Chapman, C. M. (1976). Nursing − Rhyme or Reason? *Nurs. Times* 72, Suppl., 109−12.

Cheadle, J. (1971). Three weeks in the life of a psychiatric charge nurse. *Nurs. Mirror* 133, 39−42.

Cordiner, C. M. (1968). Personality testing of Aberdeen student nurses. *Nurs. Times* 64, 178−80.

Davis, B. D. (1981). The training and assessment of social skills in nursing: the patient profile interview. *Nurs. Times* 77 (15), 649−651.

Davis, B. D. and Ternulf-Nyhlin, K. (1981). The assessment of training in social skills in nursing, with particular reference to the patient profile interview. Proceedings of the Annual Conference of the Research Society of the Royal College of Nursing, University of Kent, Canterbury.

Davitz, K. J. and Davitz, J. R. (1975). How do nurses feel when patients suffer? *Am. J. Nurs.* 75, 1505−10.

Eggert, LL. (1975). Challenge exam in interpersonal skills. *Nurs. Outlook* 23, 707−10.

Farrell, M. (1977). Teaching interpersonal skills. *Nurs. Outlook* 25, 322−5.

Faulkner, A. (1979). Monitoring nurse−patient conversation in a ward. *Nurs. Times* 75, Suppl., 95−6.

Ferguson, R. S. and Carney, M. W. P. (1970). Interpersonal considerations and judgement in a day hospital. *Br. J. Psychiatr.* 117, 397−403.

Franklin, B. L. (1974). *Patient Anxiety on Admission to Hospital*. London: Royal College of Nursing.

GNC (England and Wales). Syllabus of training for the register, London.

GNC (Scotland). Schemes of training for the register, Edinburgh.

Gruen, W. (1970). Communication problems as a possible contribution to chronicity in mental patients. *Soc. Sci. Med.* 4, 307−20.

Hatton, J. (1977). Performance evaluation in relation to psycho-social needs. *Super. Nurse.* 8, 30, 32, 35.

Hays, J. S. and Larson, K. H. (1963). *Interacting with Patients*. New York: Macmillan.

Hayward, J. (1975). *Information, a Prescription Against Pain*. London: Royal College of Nursing.

Henderson, V. and Nite, G. (1978). *Principles and Practice of Nursing*. London: Collier Macmillan.

Hockey, L. (1976). *Women in Nursing*. London: Hodder and Stoughton.

Huber, C. J. and Hanson, S. (1975). Sensitivity training; a step towards involvement with patients. *Nurs. Forum* 14, 175—87.

Johnston, J. E., Rice, V. H., Fuller, S. S. and Endress, M. P. (1978). Sensory information instruction in a coping strategy and recovery from surgery. *Res. Nurs. and Hlth.* i, 4—17.

Johnston, M. (1976). Communication of patients' feelings in hospitals. *In* A. E. Bennett (ed.). *Communication Between Doctors and Patients*. Nuffield Provincial Hospitals Trust; Oxford University Press.

Jourard, S. (1971). *The Transparent Self*. New York: Van Nostrand Reinhold Co.

Kelman, H. R. (1976). Evaluation of health care quality by consumers. *Int. J. Hlth. Services* 6, 431—42.

Kerrigan, M. R. (1957). Analysis of conversations between selected students and their assigned patients. *Nurs. Res.* 6, 43—5.

Kramer, M. (1974). *Reality Shock*. St. Louis: C. V. Masby Co.

La Monica, E. L., Carew, D. K. and Windsor, A. E. (1976). Empathy training as the major thrust of a staff development programme. *Nurs. Res.* 25, 447—51.

Lelean, S. (1974). *Ready For Report — Nurse?* London: Royal College of Nursing.

Leonard, C. V. (1975). Patient attitudes to nursing interventions. *Nurs. Res.* 24, 335—9.

Levitt, R. (1975). Attitudes of hospital patients. *Nurs. Times* 71, 497—9.

Lineham, D. T. (1966). What does the patient want to know? *Am. J. Nurs.* 66, 1066—70.

Mackie, L., Alexander, M. and Grubb, M. (1979). Teaching the nursing process: revitalising the nursing care plan; adapting the nursing process for use in a surgical unit; a clinical teacher's view. *Nurs. Times 75*, 1440—9.

Malcolmson, K., Brandman, J. and Alpert, M. (1977). An evaluation of the effect of nurses wearing street clothes on socialisation patterns. *J. Psychiatr. Nurs.* 15, 18—21.

Manderino, M. A. (1977). Effects of a group assertive training procedure on undergraduate women. *Commun. Nurs. Res.* 8, 140—8.

McGee, A. (1961). *The Patient's Attitude to Nursing Care*. Edinburgh: Livingstone.

Menzies, I. E. P. (1960). A case study in the functioning of social systems as a defence against anxiety. *Hum. Relats.* 13, 95—121.

Miltz, R. J. (1977). Nurses improve their personal communication. *Super. Nurs.* 8, 13—15.

Moos, R. H. and Houts, P. S. (1970). Differential aspects of the social atmosphere of psychiatric wards. *Hum. Relats.* 23, 47—60.

Moult, A., Melia, and K. and Pembrey, S. A. M. (1978). *Patterns of Ward Organisation*. Edinburgh: Nursing Research Unit. Unpublished report.

Munsadia, I. D. (1971). Therapeutic effects of nurse—patient relationships. *Hlth. Bull.* 29, 73—8.

Nightingale, F. (1959—1970). Notes on Nursing; *What It Is and What It Is Not*. London: Duckworth and Co. Ltd.

Raphael, W. (1977a). *Patients and Their Hospitals*. 3rd edn. King Edward's Hospital Fund for London.

_____ (1977*b*). *Psychiatric Hospitals Viewed By Their Patients*. 2nd edn. King Edward's Hospital Fund for London.

Revans, R. W. (1964). *Standards for Morale: Cause and Effect in Hospitals*. Nuffield Provincial Hospitals Trust; Oxford University Press.

_____ (1972). *Hospitals, Communication, Choice and Change*. London: Tavistock Publications.

Rinn, R. C. (1976). Effects of nursing apparel upon psychiatric in-patients' behavior. *Percept. Mot. Skills* 43, 939–45.

Roper, N. (1973). *Principles of Nursing*. Edinburgh: Livingstone.

Ryden, M. B. (1977). The predictive value of a clinical examination of interpersonal relationship skills. *J. Nurs. Educ.* 16, 3.

Savage, B. J. and Widdowson, T. (1974). Revising the use of nursing resources 1–2. *Nurs. Times* 70, 1372–4 and 1424–7.

Sheahan, J. (1976). Education 7: Communication skills and assessment learning. *Nurs. Times* 72, 1570–2.

Singh, A. (1971). The student nurse on experimental courses II; personality patterns. *Int. J. Nurs. Studies* 8, 189–205.

Smith, C. M. (1977). Identifying blocks to communication in health care settings and a workshop plan. *J. Cont. Educ. Nurs.* 8, 27–32.

Smith, L. (1979). Communication skills: Process recordings can be used to teach psychiatry students how to communicate. *Nurs. Times* 75, 926–9.

Stewart, W. (1975). Nursing and counselling; a conflict of roles. *Nurs. Mirror* 140, 71–3.

Stockwell, F. (1972). *The Unpopular Patient*. London: Royal College of Nursing.

Towell, D. and Harries, C. (1979). *Innovation in Patient Care: An Action Research Study of Change in A Psychiatric Hospital*. London: Croom Helm.

Turner, S. (1976). Fostering personal growth through small group interaction in diploma school nursing. *J. Nurs. Educ.* 15, 37–9.

Weiland, G. F. and Leigh, H. (eds) (1971). *Changing Hospitals: A Report on The Hospital Internal Communications Project*. London: Tavistock Publications.

de Wever, M. K. (1977). Nursing home patients' perception of nurses' affective touching. *J. Psychol.* 96, 163–71.

Wilson-Barnett, J. (1979). *Stress In Hospital: Patients' Psychological Reactions to Illness and Health Care*. London: Churchill Livingstone.

de Wolfe, A. S., Barrell, R. P. and Cummings, J. W. (1966). Patient variables in emotional response to hospitalisation for physical illness. *J. Consult. Psychol.* 30, 68–72.

Wolfer, J. A. and Davis, C. E. (1970). Assessment of surgical patients pre-operative emotional condition, and post-operative welfare. *Nurs. Res.* 19, 402–14.

3 Doctor–patient skills

PETER MAGUIRE

Introduction

When a patient seeks medical help the doctor's first task is to ensure that he behaves in a way which leads the patient to trust him and disclose why he has presented, otherwise the doctor may not determine the true nature and extent of the patient's current difficulties. Once the doctor has made a diagnosis he has to discuss this with the patient and explain any action he plans to take. Unless he does this adequately the patient will probably feel dissatisfied and fail to comply with advice or treatment.

The patient may be extremely worried about the possible diagnosis, investigations and treatment. His fears can be allayed only if the doctor is able to clarify exactly what they are and reassure him. The history, physical examination and investigations may reveal a potentially life-threatening or fatal illness. The doctor has then to decide whether, when and how to break the news to the patient and close relatives. Failure of the doctor to correctly identify what they wish to know about the disease and prognosis may hinder their attempts to cope and lead to serious psychological problems. Doctors can discharge these important tasks effectively only if they possess the relevant skills. Unfortunately, many do not appear to acquire them during their professional training.

Deficiencies in history-taking skills

Medical students

Studies of medical students have found that they experience considerable difficulty when obtaining a history of patients' presenting complaints and commonly fail to explore relevant psychological and social aspects (Maguire and Rutter 1976). Direct observation of interviews conducted by fifty senior medical students found that these difficulties stemmed from a lack of certain essential skills.

Each student was asked to obtain a history of the present illness or problems from a patient previously unknown to them. They were allowed fifteen minutes for this and told that they should try to end their interviews on time. This time limit was imposed because it approximated much more closely to the time they would have when qualified than the hour or more they were usually allowed for interviews. Only those patients who were likely to be helpful to the students were chosen. All of these were recovering from a depressive illness or an anxiety state. Students were informed that the aim was to establish their level of interviewing skills and that this would be done by recording the interviews on videotape and rating them.

Subsequent analysis showed that the students lacked essential skills. 86 per cent were too willing to accept data from their patients that were very imprecise. Consequently, they failed to establish when the patients' problems had begun or the relation between these problems and factors which may have triggered them. They were similarly vague about any treatments the patients had received, even though most patients would have told them if asked the appropriate questions. Almost as many (80 per cent) were noticeably reluctant to ask about patients' marriages, other personal relationships, social life and sexual adjustment even when these were relevant to a proper understanding of their problems. When patients spontaneously raised such matters, as most did, the students seemed not to hear them or tried to move them on to more neutral topics.

Most patients used medical jargon when describing their presenting complaints. Few students (8 per cent) attempted to clarify just what the patient meant by words like 'anxiety', 'heartburn', 'depression' and 'diarrhoea'. Consequently, many students gained a false idea of what was wrong with their patients. Most patients gave several clear verbal clues about the nature of their presenting complaints within the first few minutes of the interview. For example, one patient mentioned that she had been experiencing 'pains in my chest', feeling 'out of sorts' and 'sleeping poorly'. The student concentrated on her descriptions of pain and proceeded to clarify these. Although the patient often repeated that she had felt 'out of sorts' and had been 'sleeping poorly' he continued to focus on her pains. Consequently, he failed to realize that her main problem was a depressive illness and not her chest pains, which had no organic basis.

Shortage of time is often given by doctors as a reason for their failure to identify their patients' problems. It was striking, therefore, that 72 per cent of students wasted much of the available time through unnecessarily covering the same topic several times. Even when the students successfully obtained the relevant information it was often confused and contradictory. This was partly due to the students' reluctance to clarify just what the patients meant. When one woman mentioned she had been suffering from diarrhoea the student assumed she meant loose, runny stools and attributed it to the anxiety she was also experiencing. However, her anxiety was due to her observing blood and mucus in her stools.

Over half (54 per cent) of the students found it difficult to keep the patient to the point. They often allowed patients to talk at length about matters unrelated to their presenting problems despite the 15-minute time limit. When they tried to interrupt to bring the patient back to more relevant matters they did so only tenatively or half-heartedly. They seemed afraid to intervene in case they upset their patients. They often reacted to the patients they could not control by becoming restless, bored or irritated. This usually confused and upset their patients. Only 10 per cent were able to end their inter-views in the time allotted.

Only a few students (8 per cent) asked questions in a way which avoided biasing the answers they were given. Nearly a quarter (24 per cent) asked such lengthy and complex questions that patients did not know which component to respond to. Even ordinary social skills were often absent. Only a fifth of students explained exactly who they were, their status or which clinical team they were attached to. Few bothered to ensure that their patients were at ease before they began to ask questions about their main complaints or heeded indications that the patients were distressed. Some students behaved in a way guaranteed to inhibit their patients. They adopted a 'machine-gun' mode of questioning or were far too detached and disinterested. Many found it difficult to take notes and look at the patients. They were sometimes so busy writing down what was said that there was very little eye contact. Their patients got little indication, therefore, that what they were saying was acceptable and worth talking about.

The students' behaviour indicated strongly that they expected their patients to be suffering from only one main problem, whether physical or psychiatric. They generally assumed that the problem was more likely to be organic than psychological despite the psychiatric setting in which they were conducting their interviews. Very few students followed a predictable sequence of questions, apart from those directed at a review of the major physical systems of the body. Nor was it possible to discern any consistency in the way they began, conducted or terminated their interviews. There was often little connection between consecutive topics and it seemed more often a matter of chance which areas they covered. Only rarely did they try to establish how any problems had affected the lives of their patients and their families.

Similar deficiencies were found by Helfer (1970) when he used simulated parents of sick children to assess the interviewing skills of senior medical students. He noted that they used techniques which hindered the collection of relevant information, relied on leading questions, used unfamiliar medical jargon, cut off patients' communications and neglected to pursue important psychological and social aspects.

Junior hospital doctors

When 145 interns and residents were observed while they conducted 15-minute interviews and physical examinations a similar pattern of problems was noted. Patients were asked too many questions and not allowed to tell their stories in their own way. Consequently, they were reduced to giving monosyllabic answers to direct questions. Attempts at clarification were few and the onset, cause and precipitants of the key complaints were rarely established. The doctors commonly ignored any questions asked by the patients (Weiner and Nathanson 1976). Studies of general medical patients have suggested that junior doctors usually avoid asking them questions about their mood, reactions to their illness or its effect on their families.

Experienced hospital doctors

When Korsch, Gozzi and Francis (1968), used audiotape recordings to monitor a series of over 800 consultations between paediatricians, sick children and their mothers they found a considerable number of deficiencies. Only 24 per cent of mothers believed that they had been able to mention their real worries about their child during the consultation. Although they had usually tried to do so, the doctors appeared uninterested and failed to realize what the mothers were attempting to disclose. Most mothers, therefore, gave up trying.

Over half the doctors used complicated medical words which the mother did not understand. They wasted much unnecessary time through needless repetition or getting into unhelpful battles with the mother. Many even failed to introduce themselves before they asked questions and a substantial proportion were perceived by the mothers as cold and uncaring.

This failure of doctors to respond to cues given by patients or relatives about their main concerns was also found in a study of communications between surgeons and women attending a breast clinic. Although most (95 per cent) of those who had rated themselves as very distressed on a self-rating scale just before the consultation gave clear verbal or non-verbal clues that they were upset, these were heeded and clarified in only 5 per cent. In 20 per cent of cases the surgeons appeared to have realized that the woman was worried but dealt with it by bland general statements such as 'Don't worry, there's nothing to be bothered about' or 'We'll sort it all out for you'. In the remaining 70 per cent there was no evidence that they had picked up the cues. Only rarely did any of the surgeons enquire directly about how the women had reacted emotionally to the discovery of breast disease and possible cancer. Consequently, many of those who had been distressed before the clinic were just as distressed afterwards (Maguire 1976).

This failure of doctors to enquire systematically how patients and relatives are adapting psychologically and socially to serious physical disease may partly explain why so much of the associated psychiatric morbidity remains hidden. In a recent study of patients who underwent mastectomy for cancer of the breast, the surgeons detected only a fifth of those who had developed psychiatric problems. They also commonly failed to realize the extent to which women were suffering pain, swelling and disability in the arm affected by surgery or adverse physical toxicity when treated with cytotoxic drugs (Maguire, *et al*. 1980a).

General practitioners

General practitioners often argue that they are in the unique position of 'knowing' their patients and there is little risk of missing any physical or psychiatric morbidity which presents to them. However, direct observation of general practice found a wide variation in the ability of individual practitioners to detect psychiatric illness (Marks, *et al.* 1979). Some identified as few as 20 per cent of those affected while others recognized as many as 80 per cent. Importantly, there was a strong correlation between their detection rate and the use of certain history-taking techniques. Those who asked their patients about their families, and how they were getting on at home and also asked questions designed to elicit the presence or absence of psychiatric symptoms and were responsive to verbal cues had a much better recognition rate. This ability to recognize problems was not related to the amount of time the GPs spent in consultation.

Other broader and larger observational studies of general practice have claimed that many doctors use an inflexible style of history-taking and do not respond to the varying needs of different patients. They tend to focus on the first symptom offered and do not bother to probe any further. They seem unwilling or unable to enter into any real relationship with the patient and seek to prevent or stifle any expression of feeling (Byrne and Long 1976). Although many patients 'offer' their problems to their GPs, the GPs miss most of these and are sometimes so controlling that they stop patients talking as soon as they are about to say anything significant. They often seem to lack an understanding of their patients' lives.

These deficiencies do not appear to be remedied by experience. Irrespective of experience, GPs are found to use few empathic statements, avoid eye contact and do not talk about personal issues. They end their consultations poorly and pay little heed to psychological and social issues (Verby, *et al.* 1979). They are especially likely to ignore psychosocial aspects when patients have established physical disease or present with physical symptoms.

When the patient presents with an obvious psychiatric problem GPs are likely to miss any concurrent physical illness. Thus in a study of 200 patients consecutively admitted to a district general hospital psychiatric unit, physical illness was diagnosed in 33 per cent. This had been recognized before admission in only half of these cases (Maguire and Granville-Grossman 1968). This suggests that GPs, in common with other doctors, assume that patients will have either a physical or a psychological problem. Once they have decided which it is likely to be they cease to probe for the other type.

These studies of medical students and doctors clearly show that there is a consistent lack of certain key history-taking skills which is not compensated for by greater experience or postgraduate training.

Lack of skills in the exposition

There has been much less study of the ways doctors give patients information and advice about their disease and treatments. Even so, there is considerable indirect evidence that many doctors are equally deficient in these skills.

Surveys of patients in hospital and the community reveal that many feel dissatisfied with the amount of information they are given about their condition and treatment. They commonly complain that they did not understand what their doctor said to them and had insufficient opportunity to ask questions and discuss any worries. In a study of general practice only 18 per cent of social class 1 and 6 per cent of social class 5 patients said that their doctors were good at explaining things to them. In hospital studies the proportion expressing dissatisfaction with the information given has ranged from 5 to 65 per cent (Ley 1977).

In view of these findings it may not be surprising that, on average, 50 per cent of patients fail to comply with medical advice and treatment. For example, even insulin, which could be life-saving for diabetics, was found to have been taken in the wrong dose by half of them. Moreover, 34 per cent had no knowledge of how to test their urine and so had no proper basis on which to estimate the dose. Poor compliance with advice and treatment has been linked to perception of the doctor as business-like rather than warm and friendly, neglect of psychological and social aspects of illness, lack of feedback from the doctor, poor explanation of diagnosis and failure to meet patients' expectations. It represents a major problem in medical practice, since it renders much of the offered treatment and advice ineffective.

Inadequate preparation for major investigative and surgical procedures

These deficiencies in the explanations given to patients have been especially apparent in patients undergoing major investigations or surgery. They have complained that they were not given enough information beforehand and that this made them much more fearful than they would otherwise have been. It has caused some patients to claim that they would not have agreed to surgery had they fully realized what it entailed. Inadequate preparation has been commonly given as an explanation by patients who fail to adapt psychologically to major surgery such as mastectomy or colostomy.

Doctors find it especially difficult to communicate with patients who are diagnosed as having cancer. There is commonly a serious mismatch between the patient's wish for information and the doctor's willingness to provide it. Many doctors still take refuge in a set of rules such as 'I tell those I believe can take it and don't tell the others'. Their decision about whether or not to share the diagnosis with the patient then depends on their judgment of the patient's capacity to cope rather than on the patient's own wishes, even when these are openly expressed. Thus when one doctor was asked 'Have I got cancer?' by a patient, he elected to lie and say no. He justified this by saying 'I did not think he really wanted the truth − I am sure he wanted to believe he was all right'. Ironically, the patient had already realized that he had cancer, through talking to other cancer patients on the ward. He had given several obvious clues that he knew but these were ignored. Doctors may also go against the patient's wish to know by agreeing with the relatives' request that they should not be told.

Difficulties in communicating with the dying and bereaved

Studies of patients dying in hospitals or at home have found that many of their problems continue unabated because they are not recognized by their doctors or disclosed by the patients. Even problems like nausea, breathlessness, pain, anxiety, depression and mental confusion, which cause much distress to patients and relatives, are often unknown to the doctors (Cartwright, *et al.* 1973). There has been little systematic study of how doctors relate to the recently bereaved. However, it seems likely that they often feel inadequate when called upon to do so, especially when faced with strong feelings of sadness or hostility and when they feel upset by the death.

Why skills are inadequate

Inappropriate methods

Most medical schools and postgraduate training programmes continue to rely on the time-honoured apprenticeship method. Medical students and trainees learn through a series of attachments to different consultants or general practitioners. They are expected to observe them at work as well as interview new and old patients on their own to establish their key complaints.

Their skills in taking histories are usually judged on the basis of their written or verbal reports which they present in seminars or on ward rounds. And yet the way they perform in these settings often bears no relationship to how they related to their patients. It is most unlikely, therefore, that any deficiencies in their history-taking skills will be brought to light and remedied. In these circumstances students will probably not show much gain in their skills, and this has been confirmed in recent studies. Students taught to take psychiatric histories by the apprenticeship method failed to improve their skills (Maguire, *et al.* 1978).

While methods used to teach history-taking skills are clearly inadequate, this is even more true of the approaches used to teach the giving of advice and information, the preparing of patients for investigation and surgery and communicating with seriously ill patients, the dying and the bereaved.

Inappropriate model

At the beginning of their work with patients students are usually given printed handouts to help them learn the questions they must ask to elicit their patients' physical complaints. These do not often include items designed to help them elicit social or psychiatric problems. Nor do they include detailed discussion of the techniques which the students should use to put their patients at ease and encourage them to disclose their problems. Instead, it seems to be assumed that students already know how to begin and end their interviews, even though they are not normally expected to limit the time they spend with patients to that which will be available when they qualify. It is also assumed that they can establish good rapport, keep patients to the point, pick up and clarify verbal and non-verbal cues, avoid jargon and probe about more personal matters.

When teachers discuss history-taking they heavily emphasize the questions about physical illness. Most neglect psychological and social aspects and may actively discourage their students from probing in these areas. Their emphasis on organic illness may explain Helfer's finding that medical students become less able to cover psychological aspects as they progress through medical school (Helfer 1970).

Most teachers have themselves been trained by the same apprenticeship method. They are, therefore, unlikely to realize that they are deficient in at least some history-taking skills and do not represent as appropriate a role model as they would like to believe. Nor will many of their students realize this. If they are later presented with more appropriate models by psychiatrists or general practitioners they are likely to reject them because they differ considerably from those originally presented. Even when more useful models of history-taking are offered they do not often include discussion about how to assess information needs, provide information and advice. Instead, students usually have to deduce the best methods from watching the 'experts' at work.

Few 'experts' appear to be aware of the considerable literature on factors that enhance patient comprehension, recall, satisfaction and compliance. Thus, when they talk to patients about their condition they pay little if any heed to the value of giving the most important information first, presenting different kinds of information separately, limiting the amount of data given and clarifying the patients' perception and attitudes about their problem (Ley 1977). They often overestimate the patient's knowledge of anatomy and commonly use medical terms, but underestimate their knowledge of disease and treatment. Thus few students are given an appropriate example of how best to communicate with their patients; more commonly they will be exposed to teachers who spend little time giving patients information and advice and prefer to stand at the end of the patients' beds when talking about them.

Doctors' preparation of patients for major investigation and surgery also often neglects the need to first clarify what patients know or fear about what is to happen. Instead, patients' attempts to broach their worries through statements like 'I'm frightened I'll not survive the anaesthetic' are usually met with bland reassurances that there is no risk.

The lack of effective role models is even more evident in the area of communicating with the seriously ill, especially cancer patients. Students and trainees are usually presented with dogmatic rules about telling and not telling. They are only rarely shown how to establish what such a patient desires to know. Few students are given guidelines about how to talk with patients who are dying, or the bereaved. Indeed the more complex and demanding the skills and understanding required, the less likely they are to have been taught them. These deficiencies in the training offered by most medical schools have been evident for some time. It is, therefore, worth considering why training in these skills has been neglected.

Reasons for neglect

Doctors are assumed to possess these skills

Many doctors believe that they already possess the necessary skills in communication. They argue that this must be so because most of their patients appear well satisfied with the care they give. However, this view ignores factors that commonly prevent patients from expressing any dissatisfaction directly to their doctors.

Patients are clearly dependent on their doctor for advice and treatment. If they complain the doctor may perceive them as ungrateful and give them a lower standard of care than he would otherwise have done. He might even refuse to offer any further treatment and suggest that they consult someone else. Moreover, doctors are usually extremely busy. Patients are loath to take up valuable time on complaints lest the doctor neglects the problems they want help for.

Many hospital consultations are conducted in crowded clinics where the conversation can be overheard by other staff or patients. This can be especially inhibiting to patients who are considering whether or not to voice any dissatisfaction. Even if they are interviewed in more privacy, other medical and nursing staff are usually present. Consequently, patients often feel outnumbered and at a considerable disadvantage. Most doctors come from middle-class backgrounds. Patients from less advantaged backgrounds may feel diffident about complaining because they feel there is a social distance between them and the doctors and have difficulty finding the right words.

When patients do try to complain directly, it is such an uncommon event that the doctor may take it personally and react with hostility. More commonly he will try to brush it aside, jolly the patient out of it or justify his behaviour, as in the following example:

A 45-year-old single woman felt extremely bitter when she believed she had been unnecessarily persuaded to have a breast amputated to remove a cancer of the breast. She expressed her feelings to the surgeon concerned who replied that he had had to perform the operation to save her life and she had been in no state to decide for herself. She found it very difficult to adapt psychologically to the loss of a breast.

It has been argued that doctors deliberately withhold information from patients to maintain their power over them. Whatever the merits of this view, few doctors appear to check systematically if their patients are satisfied with the care they are being given. Nor do they usually monitor the extent to which patients comply with their advice and treatment. Since few doctors ever receive any real feedback about their behaviour it is easy to understand why so many insist that their skills in communication are adequate; and yet this lack of feedback can have serious consequences.

In a study of women undergoing a course of drug treatment for cancer of the breast most experienced very unpleasant side effects, including depression, nausea and vomiting. Only a minority reported this to the doctors concerned. Some had feared that if they did so the drug on which their lives might depend would be reduced in dose or stopped. Others believed the side effects were inevitable and could not be treated. The lack of detailed probing by the clinicians was another contributory factory to this low rate of disclosure. Unfortunately, there was a strong link between this non-disclosure and the failure of women to complete the potentially life-saving treatment (Maguire, *et al.* 1980b).

Similarly, when the needs of dying patients were investigated by retrospective interviews with their close relatives it was found that few had mentioned problems with confusion, anxiety or depression, because they believed that there was little the doctor could do to relieve their suffering (Cartwright, *et al.* 1973).

Doctors cannot acquire them

Even when doctors accept that there could be some deficiency in communication skills within the medical profession they usually exempt themselves. They believe that 'You were either born with them or you were not' — these are not the kinds of skill that can be learned; deficiencies cannot, therefore, be remedied. Yet there is now considerable evidence that many of these skills can be taught.

Students who were asked to practise interviewing patients under conditions of a strict time limit and videotape recording and then given feedback about their performance showed a substantial gain in several essential interviewing skills. These included the ability to pick up and clarify verbal leads, help the patient keep to the point (control) and ask about more personal but relevant matters such as marriage, sexual adjustment and the possibility of suicidal ideas (Maguire, *et al.* 1978).

A similar acquisition of skills occurred when beginning medical students were shown videotapes demonstrating how to interview and then given a chance to practise them systematically (Maguire, *et al.* 1977). Feedback techniques have also proved of considerable value in teaching interviewing skills to general practitioners. More personal qualities such as the ability to convey that you understand how the patient feels about his predicament (empathy) have also been taught successfully (Poole and Sanson-Fisher 1979).

While it is already clear that interviewing skills can be learned through more effective methods of training, the extent to which the skills used in giving advice and information can be taught has yet to be established. Similarly, although there have been attempts to teach communication with cancer patients, the dying and bereaved, these have yet to be properly evaluated.

Using these skills will create problems

The practice of clinical medicine is a stressful occupation. Doctors continually deal with the seriously ill, chronically disabled and dying and are ultimately responsible for the care of their patients. Their reluctance to accept the need for training in communication skills may be linked to their need to survive these pressures.

If they communicate effectively with their patients they are going to be confronted with the emotional effects of the illness, their advice and treatment. For example, a doctor whose work includes the treatment of leukaemia has to use extremely unpleasant drugs to try to eradicate the disease. These may cause enormous suffering to the child and his or her parents. If the doctor tries to consider such effects he may feel upset and question the advisability of continuing treat-ment. He also knows that if he stops treatment the child will die. If he specializes in this area he will have to treat many such children and will often encounter this dilemma. How often can he afford to be upset in this way?

He will also have to come to terms with the fact that many of these children will die. If he has established a good rapport with a child and family and communicated effectively with them he will be likely to experience the child's death as a personal loss. How many losses can he suffer and yet continue to be effective in treating children with leukaemia?

Doctors confronted with such potentially distressing situations may unwittingly distance themselves from the effects of illness and treatment. They may do this simply by not asking questions about them. Instead, they focus on the physical well-being of the child and assume that unless the patient or relatives complain all must be well. This need to survive emotionally may also account for doctors' reluctance to probe about psychological and social aspects of disease. Doctors and medical students readily acknowledge that they feel inadequate when called upon to ask patients about their marriage and sexual adjustment or pursue the possibility of psychiatric or interpersonal problems. They find it difficult and taxing to break the news to patients who have a potentially fatal illness or are dying. Patients who express considerable anger, bitterness or despair also provoke much unease and uncertainty in the doctor. Patients who refuse to accept the doctor's advice, suffer from chronic disability, are worried about their illness but have a trivial problem, who are adolescent, or present with their spouse are recognized as arousing considerable anxiety in the doctor (McNamara 1974, Bennet, *et al.* 1978). It would be surprising if students and doctors did not try to avoid these more demanding situations.

The skills are assumed to have no important effect on care

When faced with the evidence that many skills in communication can be taught effectively some medical educators still question the need for such training. They argue that these skills have no important effect on the care given to patients or its outcome, and there is some justification for this view.

Over the past decade many teachers have described the introduction of courses in communication skills and claimed that they are effective. However, few have attempted to establish that the use of these skills has any effect on their clinical practice. Thus on common-sense grounds teachers may argue that the ability to pick up verbal cues from patients and clarify them are important skills and should be taught; however, their use may not affect the adequacy of diagnoses, patient satisfaction, compliance and adaptation to major investigations and surgery.

Although those who advocate the teaching of communication skills need to make more effort to determine the validity of particular skills some progress has already been made, particularly with history-taking and interviewing skills. Senior medical students who acquired history-taking skills through systematic practice and feedback of performance were able to obtain much more accurate and relevant information about their psychiatric-patients' problems than students who did not learn these skills (Maguire, *et al.* 1978). Since the history alone allows doctors to establish the true diagnosis in 83 per cent of medical patients the potential importance of this improvement in history-taking ability is obvious (Hampton, *et al.* 1975). The students may have gained their additional information by behaving in ways which upset the patient. For example, they might have adopted tough interrogation methods. However, when medical students were taught these skills at the beginning of their training by watching demonstration videotapes and practising history-taking, those who used the desired skills were perceived by the patients as more likeable, empathic and effective than those who did not (Maguire, *et al.* 1977).

While training medical students in history-taking skills leads to more accurate diagnosis and greater patient satisfaction in the short term, it is not yet clear whether these effects last or if they are generalized to other settings than the one in which the students were taught. Thus the students may apply these skills when they know they are being observed but fail to do so when they are not observed. They may practise them while doing a clerkship in psychiatry but not use them at all in subsequent clerkships in general medicine or surgery. Work by Poole and Sanson-Fisher (in press) found that students who had been taught how to be empathic 3 years earlier showed a definite decline but were still considerably better than students not taught this skill. This suggests that training in communication skills ought to continue throughout their clinical years.

A recent study by Goldberg, *et al.* (1980) has been especially encouraging. They set out to teach American trainees in general practice how to interview so that they could better recognize and diagnose psychiatric disturbance. They used a combination of demonstration videotapes, practice through role-play, practice with real patients and videotape feedback of performance to achieve this aim. They found strong correlations between the doctors' ability to detect psychiatric disturbance and their use of their newly acquired skills. These skills included the following: establishing good eye contact with the patient at the beginning of the consultation; the appropriate handling of case notes; the use of an appropriate degree of control to help the patients disclose their problems; helping the patient focus on the present rather than the past; clarifying verbal and non-verbal cues which patients give about their problems; and demonstrating empathy.

In another study a nurse without any psychiatric experience was trained through systematic practice and audiotape feedback of performance to use a similar range of skills to monitor the progress of women who had undergone mastectomy for cancer of the breast. She also had to be taught how to avoid blocking the patients' communications by jollying them along or trying to reassure them before she had established what was wrong with them (Maguire, *et al.* 1980a). She was subsequently able to recognize and refer for help 83 per cent of those of her patients who developed psychiatric problems. The doctors, social workers, nurses and general practitioners who were looking after an identical group of women and had not received any such training could identify only 22 per cent of those of their patients who had been similarly unable to adapt to the diagnosis of cancer, its treatment, or both. Consequently, there was four times more psychiatric morbidity in the group not followed up by the nurse.

The main focus of these studies was on psychiatric illness. The extent to which the detection of physical illness could be similarly improved by training in the relevant skills has yet to be properly determined in patients suffering primarily from physical illness. Even so, when the medical students mentioned earlier obtained more information as a result of training this applied equally to psychiatric and physical problems. Similarly, the specially trained nurse also detected more of the physically-based problems which patients developed after mastectomy. These included: pain, swelling and disability in the arm affected by surgery; recurrence of the cancer; and adverse effects of the potent drugs given to some of the women.

The emphasis on eliciting psychological aspects of patients' problems may also prove to have beneficial effects on prognosis and rehabilitation. Patients who suffer high levels of anxiety and depression are less likely to recover from their physical disease or return to a normal life-style. Attitudes to their disease and work as well as self-image may also affect recovery. For example, patients who were suffering from chronic bronchitis were much less likely to have recovered their respiratory function and returned to work if they perceived exercise as worthless and dangerous, work as dangerous and stressful and themselves as vulnerable (Rutter 1979). Training in history-taking skills could undoubtedly enable doctors to identify these attitudes better. Studies could then be carried out to determine whether these attitudes could be modified and whether this improved recovery.

There have been few attempts to train medical students and doctors systematically in the skills required to promote patients' recall and compliance with advice and treatment but the results of some experimental studies have been encouraging (Ley 1977). Four general practitioners were asked to read a manual which was designed to help them improve their ability to provide information and advice. This advised them to give instructions and advice at the beginning of the information-giving sequence and stress their importance. They were asked to use short words and sentences and present information in separate and explicit categories. For example, they should have said 'I am going to tell you: what is wrong with you; what tests will be needed; what will happen to you; what treatment you will need; and what you must do to help yourself. First, let me say what I think is wrong with you.' Their patients recalled between 61 and 80 per cent of the information given by their doctors when they used these methods. This was significantly more than the 52–59 per cent of data they recalled when these methods were not used.

Better comprehension and recall should lead to better compliance, and there is some support for this view. Women who wished to keep to a low-carbohydrate diet were given a leaflet which was either very easy or moderately easy to read and understand. The simpler leaflet resulted in more weight loss. A similar effect was found when 160 psychiatric outpatients were given one of three leaflets giving them information about the antidepressants or tranquillizers they were to receive. The leaflet that was most difficult to read was typical of those often given. The other two were especially designed to be easy or moderately easy to read. Compliance was assessed on the basis of pill counts. The 'difficult' leaflet was ineffective in promoting compliance but medication errors were much fewer in patients given one of the other leaflets.

These studies suggest that doctors could substantially improve recall and compliance if they avoided presenting information in a complex or difficult form, realized that most patients lack elementary technical knowledge and checked to see whether the patient had any misconceptions. Claims that doctors who are friendly, clarify patients' views and expectations about their disease and treatment, and spend time talking about non-medical matters obtain greater patient satisfaction and compliance still need to be tested experimentally.

Preparation for major investigation and surgery

The systematic provision of information and support to patients who are to undergo surgery or special investigations appears to have beneficial effects (Ley 1977).

Egbert, *et al.* (1964) compared a control group who received only the care routinely given with patients who were also told what pain to expect, given instruction about postoperative exercises and visited more regularly by the anaesthetist. The experimental group recovered sooner, required fewer analgesics and was discharged earlier. In another study Schmitt and Wooldridge (1973) compared the effects of routine preoperative care with those of giving information, advice and clarifying any worries or misconceptions. The experimental group were much less anxious, were discharged sooner and showed less physiological disturbance than control subjects.

These and other similar studies which have found a positive link between preoperative preparation and outcome of surgery have used several approaches at once. It is, therefore, still not clear what contributions of the ability to provide needed information and support and to clarify and correct misconceptions before surgery make to this improved outcome. Moreover, the beneficial effects have so far been shown only in relation to less serious surgery. Indeed, in a recent study of the effects of providing advice and information before mastectomy it was found that while the women welcomed this help, it did not prevent the later development of psychological and social problems (Maguire, *et al.* 1980c).

Other work has suggested that whatever approaches are used, they should be tailored to the individual needs of the patient. Patients who were experiencing low levels of anxiety were actually harmed by the presentation of a leaflet which told them about the surgical procedures which were shortly to be performed. Patients who had high levels of anxiety benefited from the leaflet (Klos, *et al.* 1980). Patients who cope by not facing the outcome of their disease and its implications may fare less well if forced to accept information. Those who cope best by knowing about what is to happen to them and why may be hindered if information is withheld. Skills in assessment are clearly required if doctors are to determine how patients best cope.

Most attempts to improve preparation of patients before surgery have relied on specially trained nurses. The extent to which surgeons and anaesthetists could acquire the relevant skills and would apply them routinely to their patients has still to be determined.

Talking with the seriously ill, dying and bereaved

Some educators have introduced courses or workshops designed to teach medical students and doctors how to communicate with seriously ill patients, especially those suffering from cancer, the dying and bereaved. They have usually emphasized the use of listening skills, clarification of the patients' feelings, needs and wishes, and the importance of being alert to verbal and non-verbal cues. Without rigorous evaluation of these courses it is not possible to say if they achieve their objectives and also benefit patients and relatives. However, there is no doubt that many doctors feel especially inadequate when confronted with these situations and would welcome some training.

Recent work by Hinton (1979) suggests that willingness to communicate more frankly with patients who are dying leads to a reduction in their anxiety, depression and irritability. Moreover, he found that patients preferred this openness and appeared less troubled by thoughts of dying and more prepared to discuss it than patients who had been spoken to less honestly. Attempts to counsel those bereaved people who are at high risk of developing psychosomatic or psychiatric illness have also had encouraging results (Parkes 1980). They appear to reduce the risk of a poor outcome to that of low-risk groups. Therefore, it would seem worth while to give doctors and medical students more training in the relevant skills.

The priorities of modern medicine

When some of those concerned with medical education are confronted with this case for teaching skills in communication they dismiss it immediately, arguing that the main task of the doctor is to diagnose and treat disease, especially physical illness. They consider that social and psychological problems merit much less attention because they are not based on any underlying scientific theory. From this perspective, general medicine and surgery are perceived as based on 'hard' science while psychiatry and psychology are 'soft' and, therefore, less relevant subjects. This bioengineering ideology has dominated medicine for a considerable time and led to increasing emphasis on the technology of medicine rather than the patients being treated and their families. Thus suggestions that teaching in communication skills should receive more attention are likely to be resisted on the grounds that the curriculum is already overcrowded and if any additional time is made available this ought to be allocated to general medicine and surgery.

Recently, there has been a hint that the pendulum may be beginning to swing back. Many more studies have been conducted into communication between doctors and patients and much concern has been expressed about their inadequacy. Doctors, patients and families alike have also become increasingly worried about the impairment in the quality of life that often results from modern treatments. Only systematic training in skills in communication is likely to redress the balance.

Towards more effective training

Identify deficiencies

If teachers are to properly understand the difficulties that their medical students and doctors experience in attempting to communicate with patients it is important that they first identify the exact ways in which they are deficient. This can most easily be done by asking the student or trainee to take a small tape-recorder with them when they are called upon to interview a patient, give information or advice, prepare patients for investigations and surgery, or talk with the seriously ill, dying or bereaved. If they explain to the patients that they wish to assess how well they communicate with them the patients will probably not object. Indeed, they are much more likely to co-operate and give the student or doctor valuable feedback about their performance.

It is usually very threatening to receive feedback about actual performance, since it exposes strengths and weaknesses which cannot be dismissed as due to the teacher's prejudice or invention. A teacher who takes the trouble to monitor how well his students perform before any training will be much more understanding of their difficulties and less critical of their performance.

Development of adequate models

Attempts to analyse deficiencies will also help in the preparation of guidelines about what the student or doctor should be trying to communicate and how they should communicate it. Such models should be quite explicit about the skills to be learned and provide clear operational definitions of them. Such specification of skills will also enable performance to be properly assessed.

Measurement of performance

If training is to be effective teachers must be able to assess performance reliably. They can do this accurately only if they have received some training in the use of appropriate rating scales or rely on ratings made by others.

The simplest approach is to use global rating scales to assess the extent to which students or doctors use specified skills during an encounter with a patient. Thus a five-point scale (0—4) was used to assess medical students' ability to respond to verbal cues. A score of '0' meant that they showed no ability to respond to verbal cues, while a score of '4' indicated that they were extremely good at this. Raters using such scales were able to obtain a high level of agreement about a student's performance. They also maintained their own rating standards over time (Maguire, *et al.* 1978).

Simpler skills, such as introducing oneself by name, could only be rated as present or absent and ratings of these were almost totally reliable. Although this type of rating system can be learned easily by teachers, its validity has not been determined. Thus it is not yet clear how well such global ratings validly reflect the number of times the student or doctor used particular behaviours.

Other teachers have preferred to assess performance by analysing each item of behaviour and classifying it as belonging to one of a series of predetermined categories. They have usually based such judgments on transcripts of the interview. However, simplified versions have been developed which can be completed as the interview proceeds. Thus the observation schedule developed by Morrison and Cameron-Jones

(1972) for use in general practice included the following ten items: salutation, reassurance, invitation/initiation, encouragement, command, direct question, problem resolution, symptoms, problem-related expression and questioning. They were able to construct profiles for each trainee on how often they used each of these categories of behaviour. Byrne and Long (1976) also favoured this approach and distinguished between behaviours which were doctor centred, patient centred or negative. Both the global and item-analysis approaches offer students and doctors reliable measures of their performance and affects of training. No direct comparison has yet been made of the two approaches in terms of their effects on the learning of skills.

Method of training

The first decision a teacher must make is how best to present the skills to be learned. Merely presenting printed handouts can be effective but using television to demonstrate the skills in action is likely to be more so. If teachers have the necessary resources to make their own material they may wish to do so. Alternatively, they may wish to use videotapes made for more general distribution. For example, the Association of University Teachers in Psychiatry has produced a series of tapes which demonstrate basic interviewing skills. Such tapes may illustrate the use of the correct skills (modelling) or discuss the advantages and disadvantages of using other behaviours. They can be presented to large groups or watched individually by medical students or doctors.

Once the mode of presenting the desired skills has been decided the teacher has to determine how best to help the student or doctor acquire the skills. It is crucial that the trainee has a chance to practise the desired skills and is directly observed while doing so. Since direct feedback by a tutor about performance is relatively ineffective the practice of skills should be recorded on audiotape or videotape. The trainee can then see for himself exactly how he performed.

The tasks set the trainee should approximate closely to those which he will meet in clinical practice. Thus, if he is going to have only five minutes available for consultation it is important that at some stage he is given only five minutes to see how he handles such time limits. Some teachers may prefer to begin by asking trainees to practise only one skill at a time and limiting discussion to that (microcounselling).

Others present trainees with a whole group of skills to be practised. Both are effective but it is not clear if either method is superior to the other. It could also be that some skills are easier to learn than others. It would then be sensible to teach these first.

Practice conditions

Trainees may practise with other trainees or the teacher (role–play), with real or simulated patients. The advantage of simulators is that the level of complexity of the problems they present can be matched to the trainees' training needs and they can give valuable feedback about how they felt the trainees went about their task. They also avoid the risk of exposing real patients to unskilled trainees. This may be especially important when attempting to teach the skills of communication with the seriously ill, dying and bereaved (Sanson-Fisher and Poole 1980).

Despite the attractions of using simulators there could be disadvantages. Students and doctors may learn less efficiently than if they practise with real patients and the simulators could conceivably be harmed by their experience. While studies are needed to clarify these issues, training could combine all three methods. Trainees could begin by clarifying the desired skills through role play and then progress to practise with simulated patients. Finally they could practise with real patients.

Mode of feedback

Feedback via television or audiotape replay both result in significant learning of interviewing skills but audiotape recording and replay is the much cheaper method. It would seem sensible, therefore, to use audio-recording to help students and doctors achieve a reasonable level of skill. Videotape recording and replay could then be used to sharpen up these skills and focus on non-verbal behaviours.

Attempts to encourage students as individuals or in small groups to teach themselves through watching videotape replays have proved disappointing (Maguire, *et al.*, unpublished observations). They learned much less than students who were given feedback individually or in small groups by a supervisor. The presence of a supervisor enables trainees to understand better the skills being taught and realize what their strengths and weaknesses are. It also leads to them enjoying training more.

Since the provision of individual feedback is time consuming it is encouraging to find that when students are taught in small groups of four they fare as well as when taught individually by a supervisor, even though only one of their interviews is discussed on each occasion. Therefore, training large numbers of medical students or doctors through systematic practice with real or simulated patients and then giving them audio-feedback of performance within small groups in the presence of a supervisor is workable.

Who should teach

Most attempts to formally teach skills in communication have been made by interested individuals or departments. Some medical schools have invited behavioural scientists, especially clinical psychologists, to mount special courses, usually in the preclinical years or during the students' introduction to clinical medicine. In other schools, departments of medicine, paediatrics, general practice or psychiatry have carried the burden of such teaching. Rarely has more than one department been involved in any medical school.

These attempts have usually been effective in the short term but they suffer from several disadvantages. As long as the need to train in these skills is propounded by a minority of departments, students may see them as being of limited importance. Their newly acquired skills may decline during subsequent training, especially if when they try to use them they are discouraged from doing so. They may try to use them only when they talk with the kinds of patients they originally practised with.

Similar disadvantages usually apply when the training is carried out by departments which have been specially created to teach skills in communication, for the students practise in these departments using role play and simulators rather than in the outpatient clinics or on the wards. If these departments were given sufficient personnel and resources they could attempt to integrate their teaching with that carried out by the clinical teams. They could also have access to the students at several points during their training and move from simple to more complex skills.

Perhaps the most effective method would be to train ordinary medical teachers within different departments to carry out this training and to regard it as a continuing commitment. The extent to which they could and would do this has yet to be determined. However, each registrar or senior registrar who is already concerned in clinical teaching could be asked to do this. Since students are seconded to them for some weeks they could each take a group of four. Each student would be given an audiotape recorder and asked to record an interview with a patient he has been asked to see. The students could then meet for an hour with the tutor and the interview of one of the students would be discussed. The remaining three students would be advised to listen to their own tapes in the light of what was discussed. For the next three weeks the other students' tapes would each be discussed.

As the students move through their different attachments the tasks could cover history-taking, giving information, advice, preparation for investigation and surgery, and talking with the seriously ill, dying and bereaved.

Conclusion

Serious deficiencies exist in the communication skills of many medical students and doctors. Methods of training have been developed which can remedy these. The major challenges facing those concerned with teaching these skills are how to carry this out on a large scale, how to overcome the continued resistance of some medical educators and the need to demonstrate even more clearly that the skills being taught benefit patients in tangible and important ways.

References

Bennett, A., Knox, J. D. E. and Morrison, A. T. (1978). Difficulties in consultations reported by doctors in general practice. *J. R. Coll. General Practitioners* 28, 646–51.

Byrne, P. S. and Long, B. E. (1976). *Doctors Talking to Patients*. London: HMSO.

Cartwright, A., Hockey, L. and Anderson J. L. (1973). *Life Before Death*. London: Routledge and Kegan Paul.

Egbert, L. D., Battit, G. E., Welch, C. E. and Bartlett, M. K. (1964). Reduction of post-operative pain by encouragement and instruction of patients. *N. Engl. J. Med.* 270, 825–7.

Goldberg, D. P., Steele, J. J, Smith, J. J. and Spivey, L. (1980). Training family doctors to recognise psychiatric illness with increased accuracy. *Lancet* ii, 521–3.

Hampton, J. R., Harrison, M. J. G., Mitchell, J. R. A., Prichard, J. S. and Seymour, C. (1975). Relative contributions of history-taking, physical examination, and laboratory investigation to diagnosis and management of medical outpatients. *Br. Med. J.* ii, 486–9.

Helfer, R. E. (1970). An objective comparison of the paediatric interviewing skills of freshman and senior medical students. *Paediatrics* 45, 623–7.

Hinton, J. (1979). Comparison of places and policies for terminal care. *Lancet* i, 29–32.

Klos, D., Cummings, K. M., Joyce, J., Giaichen, J. and Quigley, A. (1980). A comparison of two methods of delivering presurgical instruction. *J. Patient Counselling Hlth. Educ.* 2, 6–13.

Korsch, B. M., Gozzi, E. K., and Francis, V. (1968). Gaps in doctor–patient communications, 1. Doctor–patient interaction and patient satisfaction, *Paediatrics* 42, 855–71.

Ley, P. (1977). Psychological studies of doctor–patient communication. *In* Rachman, S. (ed.). *Contributions to Medical Psychology*. Oxford: Pergamon Press, pp. 9–42.

McNamara, M. (1974). Talking with patients: some problems met by medical students. *Br. J. Med. Educ.* 8, 17–23.

Maguire, G. P. (1976). The psychological and social sequelae of mastectomy. *In* Howells, J. (ed.). *Modern Perspectives in Psychiatric Aspects of Surgery*. New York: Bruner-Masel.

Maguire, G. P. and Granville-Grossman, K. L. (1968). Physical illness in psychiatric patients. *Br. J. Psychiatr.* 114, 1365–9.

Maguire, P. and Rutter, D. (1976). Training medical students to communicate. *In* Bennett, A. E. (ed.). *Communication between Doctors and Patients*. Oxford University Press.

Maguire, G. P., Clark, D. and Jolley, B. (1977). An experimental comparison of three courses in history-taking skills for medical students, *Med. Educ.* 11, 175–182.

Maguire, P., Roe, P., Goldberg, D., Jones, S., Hyde, C. and O'Dowd, T. (1978). The value of feedback in teaching interviewing skills to medical students. *Psychol. Med.* 8, 695–704.

Maguire, P., Tait, A., Brooke, M. and Sellwood, R. (1980a). Emotional aspects of mastectomy – a conspiracy of pretence. *Nurs. Mirror* 10 January, 17–19.

Maguire, G. P., Howat, J. M. T., Sellwood, R. A., Tait, A., Brooke, M. and Bush, H. (1980b). Psychiatric morbidity and physical toxicity associated with adjuvant chemotherapy after mastectomy. *Br. Med. J.* 2, 1179.

Maguire, P., Tait, A., Brooke, M., Thomas, C. and Sellwood, R. (1980c). Effect of counselling on the psychiatric morbidity associated with mastectomy. *Br. Med. J.* 2, 1454–6.

Marks, J. N., Goldberg, D. P. and Hillier, V. F. (1979). Determinants of the ability of general practitioners to detect psychiatric illness. *Psychol. Med.* 9, 337–53.

Morrison, A. and Camerson-Jones, M. (1972). A procedure for training in general practice. *Br. J. Med. Educ.* 2, 125–32.

Parkes, C. M. (1980). Bereavement counselling: Does it work? *Br. Med. J.* 281, 3–6.

Poole, A. D. and Sanson-Fisher, R. W. (1979). Understanding the patient: A neglected aspect of medical education. *Soc. Sci. Med.* 13, 37–43.

Poole, A. D. and Sanson-Fisher, R. W. (1980). Long-term effects of empathy training on the interview skills of medical students. *J. Patient Counselling Hlth. Educ.* In press.

Rutter, B. (1979). The prognostic significance of psychological factors in the management of chronic bronchitis. *Psychol. Med.* 9, 63–70.

Sanson-Fisher, R. W. and Poole, A. D. (1980). Simulated patients and the assessment of medical students' interpersonal skills, *Med. Educ.* 14, 249–53.

Schmitt, F. E. and Woolridge, P. J. (1973). Psychological preparation of surgical patients. *Nurs. Res.* 22, 108–16.

Verby, J. E., Holden, P. and Davis, R. H. (1979). Peer review of consultations in primary care: The use of audiovisual recordings, *Br. Med. J. i*, 1686–8.

Weiner, S. and Nathanson, M. (1976). Physical Examination: frequently observed errors, *J. Am. Med. Assoc.* 236, 852–5.

4 Psychotherapy

PETER TROWER and WINDY DRYDEN

Introduction

Psychotherapy encompasses such divergent views and practices that no one set of parameters can fully represent the topic. This presents a problem for the discussion of psychotherapy and counselling skills, since the definition of skill demands the specification of goals, procedures and criteria for success.

The problem becomes immediately apparent when attempting to define at the broadest level the nature of effective therapist skills: are these simply impersonal techniques or are they interpersonal qualities and abilities? It seems reasonable to suppose that the effective therapist needs both (Strupp 1977). He needs techniques, such as systematic desensitization in behaviour therapy or free association in psychoanalysis, which are relatively impersonal and he needs interpersonal skills,* namely those perceptual and behavioural skills used in face-to-face interaction with the client. But opinions differ greatly as to the relative contributions of technical versus interpersonal skills. For example, some psychotherapists believe interpersonal skill is the central component since, it is claimed, the therapist–patient relationship constitutes part, if not all, of the therapeutic process. Some behaviour therapists, on the other hand, believe interpersonal skills serve at best a supporting role, as a useful adjunct or facilitator of (technique-oriented) behaviour therapy, and at worst are held to be quite irrelevant to 'behavioural technology'.

Most of the evidence goes against this last, rather extreme, claim

---

* The term 'interpersonal skills' is not used in the special sense of core therapist conditions (Rogers 1957) but in the broader social psychological sense.

and indeed in the review of interpersonal skills that follows we intend to show that there is some grounds for believing that interpersonal skills, often under the guise of 'non-specific' or 'placebo' effects are just as powerful, therapeutically, as any familiar or espoused techniques. The evidence from comparative studies and surveys of such studies is certainly consistent with this view (e.g. Smith and Glass 1977). A number of these studies find that while psychotherapy of all kinds produces clear gains for clients, there are 'negligible differences in the effects produced by different therapy types' (Smith and Glass 1977). One reason for the lack of difference is the operation of relatively non-specific effects which have an influence on outcome sufficient to make additional gains from specific treatments difficult to demonstrate. Indeed the power of non-specific effects is highlighted, for example, by one study which found untrained helpers at least as effective as fully trained ones (Durlak 1979). Among the 'non-specific' variables which various authorities increasingly acknowledge as operating across all forms of treatment are the interpersonal skill variables. Even automated desensitization, once believed to be the ultimate test of technique-oriented behaviour therapy, works better if the therapist talks with a 'warm' as opposed to a 'cold' voice (Morris and Suckerman 1974). The evidence by no means settles the technical versus interpersonal issue but suggests strongly that the latter should be taken as seriously as the former, and that both should be taken as powerful components in an enlarged model of psychotherapeutic change (Shapiro 1979). In this review we shall, of course, be focusing on interpersonal therapist skills – as opposed to technical skills – and attempting to extract some of the main themes from the voluminous literature, firstly looking at the setting and some of the types of skill espoused by the main 'schools', secondly examining the empirical 'state of the art' on the most and the least effective skills, and finally examining which, if any, training methods have empirical support.

The setting

Psychotherapy is a special kind of social event, and the skills used are a function of the 'components' of the situation – the setting, the purpose, the rules and roles and so on. Psychotherapy is usually a form of face-to-face interaction using conversation between one person (or more) who is seeking help to change feelings and thoughts and behaviour, and another (or more) who is an expert providing such help. This interaction is a speech event; that is, a routinized form of behaviour delineated by well-defined boundaries and sets of expected behaviours (Labov and Fanshel 1977). The event is marked by various defining characteristics such as asymmetry — a one-way flow of self-disclosure — and these characteristics have an effect on the stylistic patterns of the therapeutic conversation. Within a single psychoanalysis session, Labov and Fanshel (1977) identified three fields of discourse with different vocalizations and rhetorical devices, which arose out of background rule and role constraints. More generally, psychotherapy may be said to deviate greatly from normal conversation, and the criteria for effectiveness in such conversation by no means necessarily apply in psychotherapy. For example, while synchrony is usually important in conversation, in psychotherapy it may not be if it is the therapist's purpose to *increase* tension or force a confrontation. The purpose of psychotherapy is different — not to enjoy a conversation or to strike a bargain, for instance, but to gain insight, to restructure beliefs and achieve other possibly painful or uncomfortable aims for the client. The effect is often the opposite of that intended in polite conversation, where weaknesses are hidden or glossed over, but in this case are highlighted instead.

The function of rules and roles of psychotherapy do vary with the rationale of the therapist's 'school'. In behaviour therapy, for example, they are supposed to provide for nothing more than a business-like relationship, but in other hands they have a central part in the process of therapy. Strupp (1977) says the therapist constantly reminds the patient of the 'basic rules' (i.e. to deal with significant, emotionally charged material) and thereby forces the patient to face uncomfortable issues.

Therapist interpersonal skills espoused by therapeutic schools

A survey of the current psychotherapies reveals a bewildering range of approaches. Although these approaches may share common therapeutic factors (e.g. mobilization of faith), they tend to differ in other ways: some use a present-time focus, others an exploration of the past; cognitive, affective and behavioural modalities of human functioning are all differentially emphasized. As we have already seen, some schools stress technical skills, whereas others emphasize the quality of the relationship and the therapist's interpersonal skills.

In this section four therapeutic approaches will be considered from the vantage point of our theme — the interpersonal skills of the therapist.

Client-centred therapy

This was founded by Carl Rogers. Human dysfunctioning is viewed in terms of the way the person has learned to ignore her own experience and has incorporated (by means of internalization and introjection) views of herself, others and the world held by significant others in her life. However, the person cannot fully ignore her experience and the resulting incongruence which often manifests itself in the discrepancy between actual self and ideal self is the basis of emotional disturbance. Rogers' belief is that it is the therapist's task to help the client reduce these discrepancies and incongruities by assisting her to value her own experience. The best way that the therapist can achieve this is by providing a certain type of therapeutic relationship. In a seminal paper, Rogers (1957) proposed a set of hypotheses which has proved the impetus for research (to be reviewed below). He argued that positive personality change in the client would ensue if the therapist:

(1) was congruent in the therapeutic hour, i.e. did not demonstrate a discrepancy between what she said and what she experienced (genuineness);
(2) experienced and endeavoured to communicate an empathic understanding of the client's expressions (empathy);
(3) experienced and endeavoured to communicate respect for the client as a worthwhile human being which was not conditional on certain client expressions or behaviours (respect), and the client perceived, to a minimal extent, the respect and empathy which the therapist endeavoured to communicate.

Studies have shown that client-centred therapists use reflection responses very often. As Patterson (1974) notes:

> Reflection responses go somewhat beyond simple acceptance responses. Reflection of content, or restating what the client is saying in different words, lets the client know that the therapist is hearing what he is saying and that he understands the content, if not what is behind it. Reflections of feelings go beyond or behind the content. They are responses to the more obvious or clear feelings that the client has about the content (p. 107–8).

These same studies show that client-centred therapists rarely direct the therapeutic process, preferring to respond to clients rather than leading them.

Although there are some technical aspects of client-centred therapy, these are kept to a minimum.* 'Reflection of feeling' has often been described as an important technique whereby the core conditions can be communicated. However, Rogers (1957) notes that 'reflection of feeling' may be made in such a way that the conditions are *not* communicated. Rogers' 1957 position was provocative in that he was proposing that these core conditions were both necessary and sufficient for change in a broad range of clients in all types of psychotherapy, not just in client-centred therapy. This early statement is still recognizable in Rogers' (1977) recent writings. However, some neo-client-centred theorists (e.g. Egan 1975) suggest further important therapist skills: immediacy, concreteness, self-disclosure and confrontation. It is difficult to tell whether these additional skills are intended as technical innovations which serve as channels for the communication of the core conditions or whether they are additional core conditions in their own right.

Psychodynamic therapy†

Although there are a number of schools within the psychodynamic tradition, there are some similarities between them. Conflicts are viewed as being acquired as a result of early experience and psychic equilibrium is maintained as long as the person's defences are operating effectively. When the defensive system begins to break down 'symptoms' emerge and the person experiences distress. It is important for the therapist to assess his client carefully before proceeding to the treatment stage. The therapist has to decide where to proceed on a supportive–uncovering therapeutic continuum (Weiner 1975). In supportive therapy, the therapist aims to help the client deal more effectively with her problems without seeking to challenge her personality style. The therapist does not delve into unconscious conflicts and often the client is helped to use her defences more

* For recent technical innovations in client-centred therapy see Wexler and Rice (1974).
† By psychodynamic therapy we are referring to the situation where therapist and client are both seated facing one another. This situation is somewhat different from psychoanalysis where the client reclines and the therapist sits out of his field of vision. The scope of this chapter is limited to face-to-face psychotherapy.

effectively. In uncovering therapy, on the other hand, the therapist aims to help the client change her personality style so that the energy which the client spends in defending her 'ego' can be released for more productive living. Here the focus of therapy is much more on uncovering the unconscious determinants of behaviour.

In both supportive and uncovering therapies, therapist interpersonal and technical skills are important. However, greater emphasis is placed by psychodynamic theorists on technical expertise. The therapist's empathy, warmth and genuineness are considered the important foundations on which the psychodynamic therapist builds (Weiner 1975). However, they are not considered sufficient for client change. In supportive therapy, although the therapist interprets materials (without challenging the client's personality style), she is also likely to offer suggestions, give advice and show herself as a close person and not as an 'as if' person in the client's eyes (Weiner 1975). In uncovering therapy, however, the position is different. Here the therapist aims to function as an 'as if' person in the person's life, strives to maintain a stance of neutrality and does not respond to the client in socially conventional ways so that unconscious motivations may be revealed by the therapist's skilful technical activity of making clarifications, confrontations and interpretations of transference and resistance material. Here the therapist's empathy, warmth and genuineness are in evidence but in a much more restrained fashion than they would be in client-centred therapy. The psychodynamic therapist, particularly in uncovering therapy, would not aim to convey warmth, for example, by markedly changing his NV pose as the client-centred therapist might. However, our effective 'po-faced' dynamic therapist is not a cold dispenser of insight-giving interventions as some more inexperienced workers are apt to interpret the neutral stance of the uncovering therapist.

Behaviour therapy

Although behaviour therapy has been defined in several ways and some now refer to the 'behavioural therapies', the behavioural approach is characterized by a number of distinguishing features:

(1) Human dysfunctioning is the result of faulty learning experiences.
(2) Dysfunctioning is maintained by antecedents and consequences both environmental and (as is now being increasingly recognized) intrapersonal.

(3) These antecedents and consequences must be specified before treatment interventions are implemented. A comprehensive understanding of these influencing variables is obtained by the therapist in a detailed behavioural analysis.

(4) Treatment goals are clearly specified and agreed upon by the therapist and client.

(5) A number of treatment techniques are used by the therapist to enable the client to reach these goals.

(6) The client learns to be her own therapist by carrying out these procedures in her own life.

Until recently, behaviour therapists had been very much technique-oriented. There are numerous studies evaluating specific procedures, but there is not much consideration of the possible mediating impact of therapist interpersonal skills on client progress. However, some behaviour therapists do, informally, show a keen awareness of interpersonal variables. Recently this issue has been addressed in the literature. Goldfried and Davison (1976), for example, present an interesting analysis of the importance of various interpersonal skills which they consider behaviour therapists should possess. They begin their analysis by stressing the importance of warm empathic interaction with clients and then continue to explore the value of the therapist's persuasiveness, her ability to create positive expectancies in clients and her ability to inspire confidence in her therapeutic procedures. Ryan and Gizynski (1971), in a study of clients' retrospective views of their experience in behaviour therapy, found that these three factors were all positively associated with behaviour change. Another acknowledged skill is the ability to structure therapy for the client. If the therapist is able to explain the behavioural orientation to human dysfunctioning to her client in ways that are meaningful to the client, present a credible rationale underlying the treatment approach, and clearly specify treatment techniques, then she has developed a working relationship with her client without which even the most powerful techniques might have minimal effect. Goldfried and Davison (1976) go further; they contend that 'the manner, style and pacing of these preparatory steps have important implications for increasing the client's motivation and enlisting her cooperation'.

This appears to be a fruitful area for the research-minded therapist's attention. A start has been made. Ford (1978) found that clients' favourable perception of the therapeutic relationship, or CPTR, in terms of therapist empathy, warmth and genuineness appeared to facilitate the process of change in assertion training, but was clearly not a sufficient basis for successful outcome. Ford (1978) suggests, however, that positive CPTR kept clients in therapy and was closely associated with short-term client change. This is reminiscent of Lazarus's (1969) argument that the core conditions of empathy, warmth and genuineness are often necessary but rarely sufficient for effecting lasting client change.

Cognitive—rational therapy

Rational—emotive therapy (RET) — founded by Albert Ellis — and cognitive therapy — founded by Aaron Beck — are two therapies of the cognitive—rational school which emphasize a direct attack on client's cognitions.* Emotional disturbance is viewed as being determined by anti-empirical thinking processes (stressed by cognitive therapy) or by the client subscribing to an irrational, demanding/catastrophizing philosophy (stressed by RET). Therapists endeavour to help clients acquire a more functional set of empirical thinking processes or a more rational preferring/anti-catastrophizing philosophy by using a wide range of cognitive, emotive and behavioural procedures.

There are similarities and differences between RET and cognitive therapy for advocated interpersonal style and skills. Cognitive therapists, usually argue that the establishment of a warm, empathic and genuine relationship with the client is essential for the working therapeutic relationship but not sufficient for lasting client change. Within the context of this empathic relationship the therapist attempts to show the client the relationship between cognitions and feelings and to teach her how she can monitor and change these cognitions. The therapist seeks to obtain the active collaboration of the client but is cautioned against overemphasizing the core conditions in the therapeutic encounter lest the client feels either undeserving of such warmth and empathy or develops an infatuation with the therapist: both situations would interfere with the desired active, collaborative relationship. Factors which enhance the

---

* A rapprochement between cognitive behaviour therapists has been in evidence in the USA recently; cognitive—behaviour therapy, the resultant hybrid, is beginning to flourish.

development of such a relationship include the therapist and client reaching a 'consensus regarding what problem requires help, the goal of therapy and how they plan to reach that goal. Agreement regarding the nature and duration of therapy is important in determining the outcome' (Beck 1976, p. 220). However, as with behaviour therapy, there is little research within the cognitive therapy framework to indicate the important influencing factors. What seems to be important is the ability of the therapist to check with the client if she understands the therapist's endeavours. Also it is important for the therapist to detect, encourage expression of and deal with the client's doubts in a non-defensive manner. Problems emerge when the therapist proceeds in a cavalier manner, paying more attention to a rigid set of therapeutic protocols rather than to the person in front of her. Beck (1976) cautions against the mechanical application of techniques and procedures without regard for the client's reactions. Goldfried and Davison (1976) make a similar point from a behavioural perspective.

While Wessler and Ellis emphasize the importance of the therapist unconditionally accepting the client, they caution against the therapist showing undue warmth towards her clients. They argue that the establishment of a warm, empathic and genuine relationship is not necessary in RET and can even be iatrogenic (causing client deterioration by therapist activities) since:

(1) It can interfere with therapy if the therapist is fearful about confronting the client because it might harm the relationship; (2) It may encourage the client to develop intense feelings about the therapist and to focus on these rather than on uncovering and disputing irrational beliefs about her outside relationships and affairs; (3) It can provide so much reassurance and direct advice-giving that the client becomes dependent on the therapist and thereby increases his/her distorted needs for love and approval (Wessler and Ellis 1979).

Ellis (1978) argues that rational–emotive therapists who have dire needs for love and approval themselves are likely to practise iatrogenic therapy as described above. While Ellis cautions against undue therapist warmth, reliable data are needed to test his hypothesis. It would be interesting to discover the optimal level of therapist warmth for effective RET. Ellis argues that the kind of relationship the active–directive, rational–emotive therapist had better strive to develop with her clients is one in which she not only unconditionally accepts clients but also serves as a good teacher, showing clients how to question and challenge, logically and empirically, their irrational beliefs. Other interpersonal skills include 'disclosing relevant facts or feelings about oneself, modelling more appropriate behaviours and the therapist thinking rationally and emoting appropriately' (Wessler and Ellis 1979). Again research is needed to determine the effect of such skills in RET with regard to manner, style of presentation and timing.

The 'effective' skills

Despite the apparent influence of schools, over 50 per cent of therapists are eclectic and disavow allegiance to any one influence and become increasingly more eclectic as they gain experience. There is, in any case, little evidence to show that therapists do what they say they do; that is, match their beliefs in an orientation to their behaviour practice. For these and other reasons most authorities now adhere to an empirical approach. In this section we examine a selection of the interpersonal skill variables which have been subjected to critical scrutiny. In some cases study of these variables emanated from schools of psychotherapy but in others emerge from quite different sources, e.g. social psychology.

In the search for effective therapist skills, investigators have been attracted to several comparatively global variables, such as the warmth—empathy—genuineness triad; power variables such as prestige, expertness and directiveness; and certain personality traits. Owing to limitations of space we can discuss only one of these variable clusters.

Empathy, warmth and genuineness

In the early 1970s Rogers' (1957) original hypothesis that the core conditions were necessary and sufficient for therapeutic outcome appeared robust. Truax and Mitchell (1971), in their review of the pre-1971 literature on this issue, claimed:

> therapists or counselors who are accurately empathic, non-possessively warm and genuine are indeed effective. Also, these findings seem to hold with a wide variety of therapists and counselors, regardless of their training or theoretic orientation,

and with a wide variety of clients or patients. Further, the evidence suggests that these findings hold in a variety of therapeutic contexts and in both individual and group psychotherapy or counseling.

However, a less optimistic picture has emerged in more recent reviews (e.g. Mitchell, *et al.* 1979, Lambert, *et al.* 1978, and Parloff, *et al.* 1978). These reviews indicate that high levels of the core conditions are only modestly related to therapeutic outcome. Even when the original hypothesis has been correctly tested − i.e. when clients' ratings are used to determine the extent to which the core conditions have been received − results do not point unequivocally to a positive association between outcome and core conditions. However, the association seems to be stronger here than when therapists' core conditions are rated by non-participant observers using taped segments.

The lack of support for the original hypothesis comes from a variety of sources. These include:

(1) The designs of most studies have not allowed for a stringent test of the hypothesis in its 'causal' form.
(2) Little relationship has been established between the ways in which the core conditions have been rated (by therapists, non-participant observers and clients).
(3) Inadequate sampling techniques have been used (e.g. of patients and therapists).
(4) Emphasis on audiotape recordings providing raw data has predominated. Here NV cues are absent. These cues have been shown to be important when empathy and the other conditions (e.g. Seay and Altekruse, 1979) are judged by non-participant observers.
(5) The scales most often used to measure the core conditions (e.g. Carkhuff 1969) may be inappropriate for schools of therapy other than client-centred (Lambert, *et al.* 1978).

Perhaps because of the last reason, lack of support for the hypothesis has been most apparent in studies using non-client-centred therapists. For example, Mintz, *et al.* (1971) in a study of fifteen experienced therapists (psychoanalytic and eclectic) found that patient outcome was judged more favourably if therapy was described as high in 'optimal empathy relationship' but seen as 'not directive'. However, if therapy was seen as 'high directive' then patient outcome was judged more favourably, when it was also described as low in 'optimal empathy relationship'.

Certain dissatisfactions have recently been expressed concerning the global nature of Rogers' original hypothesis. Lambert, *et al.* (1978) wish to know: 'Are certain therapist attitudes of particular importance at specific times in therapy?' Mitchell, *et al.* (1977) speculate that the core conditions 'might be used differentially dependent on client diagnosis'. For example, Parloff, *et al.* (1978) note that an excessively empathic statement may provoke defensiveness through heightened anxiety in some neurotics and that schizophrenic patients may not be helped, or may even be harmed, by premature therapist warmth. These questions reflect the current interest in asking specific questions about therapeutic process and outcome and merit future research.

Recently, neo-client-centred theorists have posited that certain additional therapist conditions are necessary for effective therapy. In doing so they too have expressed dissatisfaction with Rogers' original hypothesis. These theorists conceive of the therapeutic endeavour as comprising several developmental phases (e.g. Egan 1975). They argue that while therapist core conditions are important in the early phase of therapy − i.e. they help the practitioner to develop an effective, trusting, working relationship − they are not sufficient for effecting lasting client change. Other therapist skills are necessary at later stages − e.g. confrontation, immediacy and therapist self-disclosure (instigative conditions). Although some research has been carried out on these instigative conditions, few studies have been designed in the spirit of the developmentalism advocated by these theorists. An exception has been the work of Dies (1973) who has shown that the value of therapist self-disclosure is enhanced later on in therapy. These instigative conditions are considered to have potential both for client improvement and deterioration depending on whether they are offered within the spirit of a warm, empathic and genuine relationship or not. Consequently, their effects need to be studied in the context of an ongoing therapeutic relationship and not in initial interviews, as is the common practice. The conclusion of this brief overview is in agreement with the statement of Mitchell, *et al.* (1977): 'The relationship between empathy, warmth and genuineness and outcome is much more complex than had been understood earlier.'

A better way to unravel the complexities of these and other

therapeutic conditions is to take a more molecular approach: to examine the elements of therapist verbal and non-verbal behaviour and other specified skills such as perception, to examine their function during therapy and to try to relate these more precisely defined variables to outcome. We now turn to attempts in this direction.

Therapist non-verbal (NV) skills

Mehrabian (1972) and Argyle (e.g. Argyle, *et al.* 1972) have concluded from research studies that probably about two-thirds of the variability in emotion and attitude expression can be attributed to NV factors − e.g. eye contact, head-nods, body orientation, trunk lean, smiling, proximity and vocalization. One of the major problems in studying the effect of therapist NV skills has been maintaining the balance between relevance and scientific control. Much of the research in this area can be criticized for having poor external validity (the extent to which findings can be generalized to continuing therapist−client interaction). The most common paradigm includes subjects' judgments of therapist core conditions in very short, carefully prepared vignettes − ranging from single therapist−client interchanges to five-minute presentations of 'therapist' behaviour − which portrayed various patterns of therapist NV behaviours. The results of such studies have tended to support Mehrabian's (1972) conclusion.

With increasing sophistication in experimental design and data analysis, however, progress has recently been made. For example, Seay and Altekruse (1979) found that although therapist NV behaviours were important in determining client's ratings of therapist's core conditions, in only two instances (effect of trunk lean on unconditional positive regard and genuineness) did weight assumed by NV behaviour alone account for more variance than verbal style (affective and behavioural) and the interaction between NV behaviour and verbal style. Interactions were complex but tended to suggest an interesting pattern. Where therapeutic verbal style was affective (restatements of content, reflections of feeling and clarifications), increased amounts of NV activity supplemented the verbal techniques, leading to more-positive ratings. In the behavioural style (probes, interpretations, confrontations and suggestions), the more NV behaviours were used, the lower were the ratings. Seay and

Altekruse (1979) argue that the verbally active 'behavioural' therapists may have overpowered their clients if they had engaged in maximal use of NV behaviour. On the other hand, the less verbally active 'affective' therapists may have communicated lack of interest or un-attentiveness if they did not display increased amounts of NV activity. However, these findings must be interpreted cautiously. In this experiment the therapy sessions were relatively short (fifteen minutes) and therapists were inexperienced counselling trainees and although clients did present a genuine personal problem (a rare phenomenon in this group of studies), they were volunteers and may not be representative of a client sample. However, interactions were naturally occurring and not artificially created (as in other studies).

We do not yet know, with any clarity, the effect of therapist NV behaviour on client process and outcome variables in situations which resemble more closely true psychotherapy. However, such effects are probably remarkably complex.

Therapist verbal and paralinguistic skills

Research into therapist verbal style of participation is concerned with the words she uses, whereas enquiry into therapist paralinguistic behaviour is concerned with how these words are said. Paralinguistic expression consists of sounds which are not essential to the formation of words (e.g. intonation patterns, tone of voice, speech non-fluencies).

Perhaps the best example of concerted research effort in this area is the Rice—Butler—Wexler group of studies which were carried out within the client-centred framework. Results from these studies suggest that in productive client-centred therapy sessions, therapists focused on the client's inner experience using fresh, connotative language in an expressive way (Rice 1965). In addition, they sounded serious, warm, relaxed and concerned; i.e. they spoke with normal stress, oversoft intensity and overlow pitch, vocal cord control was open and when they paused, these pauses were unfilled (Duncan, *et al.* 1968). In non-productive sessions therapists' responses were within the client's frame of reference but focused on something outside the client. Commonplace language was used in most of these responses, and in more than half, voice quality was distorted (Rice 1965). Duncan, *et al.* (1968) also found that in poor sessions the paralinguistic pattern was one of forced, overloud intensity together with overhigh pitch on some occasions and oversoft intensity on other occasions. Here 'the therapist's voice would sound dull and flat, rather uninvolved, and when his voice took on more energy, he would seem to be speaking for effect — editorializing' (Duncan, *et al.* 1968, p. 567). Also when the therapist paused in these poor sessions, the pauses were filled with some phonation such as 'uh', 'um', etc. A complementary set of studies found that client expressiveness (expressive voice quality and connotative language) was significantly and positively related to therapy outcome (Rice and Wagstaff 1967) and to the level of psychological functioning (Wexler 1974). Wexler and Butler (1976), linking the research on therapist and client expressiveness, found some evidence to support the notion that a therapist could improve the poor prognosis of an inexpressive client in client-centred therapy by stimulating the client's expressive participation with the therapist's own expressive interventions.

In these studies issues were empirically addressed in a systematic way and closely related in theory. In addition genuine therapy cases were used. However, established relationships were correlational in nature and causality can only be inferred. The extent to which these findings can be generalized to other systems of therapy may be limited. They may only be specific to client-centred therapy where the primary task of the therapist is to help the client to engage in a process of self-exploration with as much freshness and immediacy as possible (Rice and Wagstaff 1967, p. 558). It is important for Rice–Butler–Wexler studies to be replicated in different therapy systems (where the therapist's primary task differs) to assess what proportion of the outcome variance can be attributed to therapist lexical and para-linguistic behaviours in therapies which place less emphasis on fresh and immediate client self-exploration as the primary mechanism for change.

Perceptual skills

The therapist can be effective only to the extent that he possesses accurate information about the client, much of which is non-verbally expressed. To achieve this he needs good perceptual skills. For example, for empathy the therapist must attend to the 'subtle non-verbal communications — the minute facial, postural, gestural clues that often contradict or multiply the meaning of another person's verbal communications' (Truax and Mitchell 1971). The therapist firstly needs to know which cues are significant and informative and secondly needs to perceive these cues without distortion by his own internal beliefs or problems. We will consider both points.

Significant information is by no means easily obtained from the defensive client. However, various studies show that the control of emotional expression leads to 'leakage' in particular microfacial and micromomentary movements, in imperfectly performed simulations of masking expression, or characteristic movements in the hands, feet and other areas which are not well monitored (Ekman and Friesen 1969). Studies also show that concealed negative feelings are leaked by repression of body movement, an increase in voice pitch, less looking and nodding, more speech errors, slower speaking rate and less-direct body orientations.

There is little research to show how well psychotherapists use this type of information. Dittman, *et al.* (1965) showed that professional dancers were significantly superior to psychotherapists in the recognition of emotional cues encoded in bodily movement. Scheflen (1965) described some of the largely unconscious quasi-courtship behaviours and their importance in psychotherapy, but these detailed observations do not seem to have been taken up. Labov and Fanshel (1977) revealed in their detailed analysis of a therapy session a number of subtle emotion cues. They observed that intense emotion is usually masked or denied but is none the less in evidence during the patient's quotations from family interaction. They included certain exchanges in intonation contour, euphemisms, vague reference, hesitation, narrative response and other indirect, complex speech acts, simple silence and omission of direct statements and simple denial of the obvious.

Even if the psychotherapist attends to the subtly revealing cues he must interpret them without undue distortion. Distortion usually occurs through cultural stereotypes and personal, 'ego-defensive' beliefs by which people interpret the behaviour of others. Therapists obviously need to guard against their own defensive perceptual tendencies more than perhaps any other professional group. Research in this area, however, reveals a depressing picture of a 'negative tendency in helpers' perceptions' (Wills 1978, p. 968) to which we return later.

The use of therapist skills in the interaction

Social interaction is a continuous process of exchanges of messages, of perceiving, interpreting and adjusting responses in the light of feedback. The skilled interactor is able to tune his responses finely in line with internal plans and external cues, and individuals differ considerably in this ability (Snyder and Monson 1975). Those high in this skill show much greater variation in their behaviour according to situational constraints than those who are low. It seems obvious that the effective psychotherapist should be high in this basic skill of using the appropriate tactic at the right time. Yet surprisingly little research has been aimed at this topic. For example, in their critical review of therapist interpersonal skills, Lambert, *et al.* (1978) ask if certain therapist skills are of particular importance at specific times in therapy – e.g. warmth at one time, empathy at another. They lament that this important topic has not been researched and suggest that 'perhaps one refinement that client-centred theory must undergo is the elaboration of the critical moments when empathy, warmth, and/or genuineness are most appropriate or helpful' (Lambert, *et al.* 1978, p. 484). They also suggest that the present practice of assigning a numeral to a complex interaction and the random sampling of segments of therapy sessions might become a thing of the past. Gurman (1977) observes that most research fails to explicate how molar 'personality' dimensions are directly and immediately manifest in therapy – i.e. what the therapist actually 'does': 'What a therapist actually does in interaction with a patient has greater impact on patient's perceptions of therapist's relationship qualities than how "expert" or "prestigious" the therapist is reputed or portrayed to be' (Gurman 1977, p. 533). Finally, Fiske (1977) similarly points out that psychotherapy research suffers the handicap of elusive, 'global' concepts which are applied to persons or behaviours, whereas what needs to be analysed are the moment-to-moment sequences of acts, such as occurs in the negotiation of speaking turns. One study showed, for example, that therapist interruptions of the patient resulted in lower perceived therapist empathy.

One way of viewing the interaction process is as influencing the patient by rewards and punishments and warmth, empathy, and genuineness variables on the one hand and power variables on the other, as skills which perhaps can be used tactically in this way. Indeed it has been shown that therapist's warmth, empathy and genuineness fluctuate during a single hour and effectiveness of, for example, empathy is probably mainly a function of it being accurately delivered at crucial moments in the session.

A number of studies on synchrony or congruence between patients and therapist suggest how patients respond to specific actions of the therapist. For example, Lennard and Bernstein (1960) found a progressive increase over four months in correlations between the percentage of therapist and patient propositions dealing with affect. Other examples of increased synchrony include 'mirror-congruent' postures and attendant increases in other patient behaviour such as self-disclosure, increases or decreases in verbal output and rate, verbal and non-verbal expressiveness and so on.

Some studies show the patient having *more* apparent influence on the therapist than vice versa, with, for example, therapist voice quality converging more towards that of the patient than vice versa, but this may simply show the therapist's greater ability to adapt and change tactics. One study showed that patients converged to the therapist more slowly than vice versa.

The interactional approach can in principle accommodate many of the apparently contradictory findings regarding, for example, the effect of therapist warmth, since it would be predicted that an effective therapist would vary his strategy according to circumstances, being consistent only with regard to the ultimate goal. The goal is not to be warm or empathic but to produce change in behaviour and attitude, for which warmth and empathy may or may not be valuable skills. A good example of this is the study by Johnson (1971) which implied that a therapist should accurately but coldly restate the patient's expressed attitude if he wants to change that attitude, and restate an attitude warmly if he wants to reinforce it.

One method of uncovering the ongoing processes is discourse analysis, as for example exemplified by Labov and Fanshel (1977). They extrapolate a number of discourse rules which enable the analyst to strip off the surface structure of mitigation and other linguistic devices to reveal the true, emotional meanings being expressed. Meanings thus embedded in various discourse forms are, of course, normally deciphered 'insightfully' by the skilled therapist but can be made explicit by this kind of analysis.

A final point in this section is to look at therapist–patient and treatment–patient interactions. Attempts have been made to match therapist and patient on personal and other characteristics to produce the best interaction and outcome. Despite considerable research effort, little convincing evidence has emerged to show what effects are due to the interaction of demographic variables, personality, value similarity, etc. Research on the well-known A–B distinction between therapist personality types and their interaction with patient types has, for example, produced almost totally disappointing results. One of the few findings is that outcome may be enhanced if therapist and patient have a similar level of differentiation of constructs but are dissimilar with regard to the content of those constructs. More promising results have been obtained with treatment–patient interaction. For example, client-centred therapy was found more effective with extroverts, rational–emotive therapy more with introverts – a finding which has implications for style preferences.

Bad therapist skills

One of the outcomes of the debate about the effectiveness of psychotherapy was the claim (Bergin 1971) that the mean response rate for psychotherapy outcome camouflaged the fact that some patients improved markedly but others deteriorated, and attention then turned to the factors responsible. Just as therapist interpersonal skills may be important in improvement, so they may be instrumental in deterioration. A number of studies confirm this.

More marked casualties seem to occur in group psychotherapy, and Yalom and Lieberman (1971) found the style of the leader was the major cause, such as the aggressive stimulator – who was the worst type. Negative effects were related to confrontation, expression of anger, rejection (by group leader), feedback overload and coercive group norms for participation.

Gurman and Kniskern (1976) showed the negative effect of focusing on emotionally loaded issues too early in therapy and of a too narrow focus on single symptoms, both in marital and family therapy. Strupp, *et al.* (1971) listed fifteen factors that led to deterioration – e.g. over-intense therapy, technical rigidity, misplaced focus and dependency fostering. Tourney, *et al.* (1966) distinguished errors of commission (therapist overactivity, including excessive probing, interruption, inaccurate and untimely interpretation, inappropriate advice and direction and provocation) and errors of omission (underactivity, including insufficient questioning and failure to provide support, interpretations and understanding). Neurotics responded to errors of commission with hostility and resistance, while schizophrenics responded with anxiety and withdrawal. To errors of omission neurotics reacted with some anxiety, schizophrenics with increased thought disorder.

Many of these negative responses can be understood in terms of countertransference — the strong feelings that the therapist may have towards the patient, and which might be unwittingly transmitted to the patient mainly by NV cues. It is widely agreed that uncontrolled countertransference has an adverse effect on therapy outcome but this seems to occur much more often than is commonly supposed (Singer and Luborsky 1977).

An example of countertransference is when the therapist is threatened by something the patient says or does, and responds defensively; that is, indulges in avoidance responses — interrupting, showing disapproval, becoming silent or ignoring the patient, thereby inhibiting patient exploration. Studies show that therapists who had problems of their own were much less accurate in perceptions of patients' difficulties in areas related to their own conflicts. Therapists who disliked their patients chose more pejorative diagnostic labels, and were rated colder and less empathic in behaviour by impartial judges.

Singer and Luborsky (1977) have developed the notion of 'negative fit' and found evidence that therapists behave in ways that conform to patients' expectations. They found two main types of 'fit' patterns: those that confirmed fear of rejection (by being critical, cold, etc.) and those that confirmed beliefs of weakness and dependence (by being domineering and controlling). Both forms were judged to be at least untherapeutic, if not antitherapeutic.

Countertransference phenomena may also account for at least some of the findings on the rather widespread unfavourable perceptions of clients by professional helpers (Wills 1978). Clients who resist influence are disliked and resented by professional helpers; helpers' perceptions of rated subjects are consistently less favourable than lay persons' perceptions, irrespective of whether the subject is normal or psychologically impaired, and experience produces an *increased* perception of maladjustment and a less generous view of clients' motivation to change; clients who are dissimilar (e.g. in social class) are liked and helped less; helpers attribute client resistance to personality defects rather than situational constraints; clinicians tend to selectively focus on weaknesses and deficiencies rather than strengths. Wills (1978) concludes that these processes operate independently of a client's adjustment problems, and in some cases work against the motivation to help.

An interesting study by Ricks (1974) provides an illustration of the negative effects of therapist countertransference reactions. Ricks studied the long-term outcome of a group of disturbed adolescents who were seen by two therapists in a child guidance clinic. Both therapists were helpful to the less disturbed boys, but when the outcome of the more seriously disturbed boys was considered a different picture emerged. The seriously disturbed boys with poor outcome were seen by a therapist who in therapy moved too soon into 'deep' material, thereby increasing feelings of anxiety in boys already experiencing high levels of anxiety. The therapist appeared to react anxiously himself to the pathology of these boys and to get caught up in their depressed and hopeless feelings, thus reinforcing the boys' sense of futility.

Therapists can not only become frightened and depressed by patient pathology, they can also use their patients to satisfy their own needs. Vandenbos and Karon (1971) call this latter phenomenon 'pathogenesis'. A study designed to assess the relationship between therapist pathogenesis and outcome in schizophrenic patients discovered that patients of more benign therapists functioned at higher levels of adjustment after 6 months of treatment than patients treated by more pathogenic therapists.

The training of psychotherapists

Before reviewing some psychotherapist training programmes, a number of sobering findings must be considered. The first point is perhaps best made by Garfield (1977) that 'the state of training cannot progress very far beyond the state of field itself. Where ambiguity and confusion reign, it is difficult to have precise, validated, and well-managed procedures'. The most critical problem, he states, concerns what is to be taught, for it is only after specifying the operations which make for positive change that we can develop and evaluate the means of teaching skills and procedures. The second point is that, despite a wealth of studies on the teaching of psychotherapy, our knowledge of effective therapist skills and training methods is, for a variety of reasons, still sadly lacking. Thirdly, for reasons no doubt embedded in the first two points, training and experience do not appear to be necessary prerequisites for effective therapy, according to recent reviews.

Paraprofessionals obtain outcomes equal to or significantly better than professionals (Durlak 1979). Furthermore, there is little information on factors that account for the effectiveness of para-professionals. Some reviewers report that professional trainees are not selected on appropriate criteria and that existing programmes are not equipping trainees with appropriate skills. It is even claimed that some clinical training schemes may actually have harmful effects upon the personalities of the students themselves. Time may show that, as with psychotherapy itself, some programmes produce beneficial effects while others may be deleterious both for client and therapist.

We shall confine ourselves to those programmes which define what is to be taught, try to relate the goals of therapy to outcome by means of valid and reliable measures, and use appropriate, research-based teaching methods. Even within this limited area, space allows for only a small sample of programmes. For more thorough coverage the reader is referred to Matarazzo (1978).

Matarazzo (1978) points out that until recently the client-centred school has provided the strongest influence towards making psychotherapy observable, its practice and training techniques specifiable, and its results measurable. They were the first to develop brief, well-formulated workshops with graded procedures. Much research has been inspired by these innovations. In accordance with the aims described earlier (p. 91), Truax and Carkhuff (1967) described the steps of the programme as follows: students were given extensive reading, followed by listening to taped individual psychotherapy sessions. They rated excerpts from the tapes on the scales of 'accurate empathy', 'non-possessive warmth' and 'genuineness'. They then practised making responses to taped patient statements. Pairs of students then role-played 'therapist' and 'patient' sessions, recordings of which were rated by supervisors on the relevant scales. After students had reached minimal levels, they had interviews with genuine patients, recordings of which were again rated by peers, the students themselves and their supervisors. After the sixth week of training, quasi-group therapy was begun with the students, who met for two-hour sessions once a week. Although subsequent research has taken the bloom off the original optimism, these training pro-grammes led the way informalizing the need for rigorous specification of skills.

Microcounselling

Ivey (1971) and his co-workers also exemplified the trend to break up complex skills into components. A recent version of this approach is as follows:

(1) A five-minute segment of therapy is videotaped.
(2) A written manual describing the single skill being taught is presented to the trainees. Video models of an expert therapist or example of a good communication illustrating the skill are shown. Trainees view their own videotapes and compare their performance with the written manual and video model. The supervisor provides didactic instruction and emotional support.
(3) A second therapy session is videotaped.
(4) The second session is examined, and the whole procedure is recycled if necessary to bring the trainees' performance up to the required level. About an hour is required for a single cycle.

Cue discrimination, modelling procedures and operant reinforcement are used throughout, with particular attention given to NV behaviour. The programme covers a number of skills, including attention, accurate reflection and summary of feeling.

Behaviour modification

Specificity is one of the hallmarks of the behaviour modification approach, and training programmes have been developed for particular professionals − such as parents, teachers or nurses − and for particular settings, clients and problems. An example of one of the more general applications for training therapists in a behavioural orientation is that of Levine and Tilker (1974). They propose gradual exposure of the student through the following steps:

(1) Non-participatory observation.
(2) Role playing to develop information-gathering skills.
(3) Sitting in on an interview, followed by a discussion with the supervisor. Initially the interview is conducted by the supervisor, and at a suitable point roles are reversed.
(4) Use of the 'bug in the ear' device, enabling *in situ* instruction and feedback, with the student conducting the interview.
(5) Review of videotape of a whole interview session by the student.

However, there have been few attempts to devise systematic programmes for interpersonal skills *per se*. Some groups have developed perceptual and observation skills training, others have devised programmes to train staff in the systematic modification of prosocial and antisocial behaviour in institutional settings. More generally, Paul and McInnis (1974) recommend — on the basis of findings — a training focus on (1) job-related behaviour rather than general orientation, (2) concrete functions rather than abstract theory, (3) modelling and feedback rather than totally didactic presentation and (4) specified programmes based on staff—patient—setting inter-actions. Hopefully, more behavioural programmes for therapist interpersonal skills will be developed along such lines.

Personal learning

We have been primarily concerned with the effect of therapists on clients. However, social influence is reciprocal and the effect of clients on therapists has a considerable 'for better or for worse' effect on the therapeutic endeavour. Thus we consider it important for training programmes to include an element where trainees have the oppor-tunity to learn about themselves and how their strengths and their weaknesses may affect the process of therapy with different clients. Future research must determine the effectiveness of such training elements within the broader framework of psychotherapy training and indeed what forms these elements might take to promote the personal development of the therapist.

Further reading

Gurman, A. S. and Razin, A. M. (eds) (1977). *Effective Psychotherapy: A Handbook of Research*. Oxford: Pergamon Press.

References

Argyle, M., Alkema, F. and Gilmour, R. (1972). The communication of friendly and hostile attitudes by verbal and non-verbal signals. *Eur. J. Soc. Psychol.* 1, 385—402.

Beck, A. (1976). *Cognitive Therapy and the Emotional Disorders*. New York: International University Press.

Bergin, A. E. (1971). The evaluation of therapeutic outcomes. *In* Bergin, A. E. and Garfield, S. L. (eds). *Handbook of Psychotherapy and Behaviour Change*. New York: Wiley.

Carkhuff, R. R. (1969). *Helping and Human Relations*, vols. 1 and 2. New York: Holt, Rinehart and Winston.

Dies, R. R. (1973). Group therapists' self-disclosure: an evaluation by clients. *J. Counseling Psychol.* 20, 344—8.

Dittman, A. T., Parloff, M. B. and Boomer, D. S. (1965). Facial and bodily expression: a study of receptivity of emotional cues. *Psychiatry*, 28.

Duncan, S. Jr., Rice, L. N. and Butler, J. M. (1968). Therapists' paralanguage in peak and poor psychotherapy hours. *J. Abnormal Psychol.* 73, 566–70.

Durlak, J. A. (1979). Comparative effectiveness of paraprofessional and professional helpers. *Psychol. Bull.* 86, 80–92.

Egan, G. (1975). *The Skilled Helper: a Model for Systematic Helping and Interpersonal Relating*. Monterey, Cal.: Brooks-Cole.

Ekman, P. and Friesen, W. V. (1969). Non-verbal leakage and clues to deception. *Psychiatry* 32, 88–106.

Ellis, A. (1978). Personality characteristics of rational-emotive therapists and other kinds of therapists. *Psychother.: Theory, Res. and Practice* 15, 329–32.

Fiske, D. W. (1977). Methodological issues in research on the psychotherapist. *In* Gurman, A. S. and Razin, A. M. (eds). *Effective Psychotherapy: a Handbook of Research*, 23–43. Oxford: Pergamon Press.

Ford, J. D. (1978). Therapeutic relationship in behavior therapy: an empirical analysis. *J. Consult. Clin. Psychol.* 46, 1302–14.

Garfield, S. L. (1977). Research on the training of professional psychotherapies. *In* Gurman, A. S. and Razin, A. M. (eds). *Effective Psychotherapy: a Handbook of Research*, 63–83. Oxford: Pergamon Press.

Goldfried, M. R. and Davison, G. C. (1976). *Clinical Behavior Therapy*. New York: Holt, Rinehart and Winston.

Gurman, A. S. (1977). The patient's perception of the therapeutic relationship. *In* Gurman, A. S. and Razin, A. M. (eds). *Effective Psychotherapy: a Handbook of Research*, 503–43. Oxford: Pergamon Press

Gurman, A. S. and Kniskern, D. P. (1976). Deterioration in marital and family therapy: empirical and conceptual issues. Presented at the seventh annual meeting of the Society for Psychotherapy Research, San Diego, California, June.

Ivey, A. E. (1971). *Microcounseling: Innovations in Interviewing Training*. Springfield, Ill.: Charles C. Thomas.

Johnson, D. W. (1971). The effects of warmth of interaction, accuracy of understanding, and the proposal of compromises on the listener's behavior. *J. Counseling Psychol.* 18, 207–16.

Labov, W. and Fanshel, D. (1977). *Therapeutic Discourse*. New York: Academic Press.

Lambert, M. J., Bergin, A. E. and Collins, J. L. (1978). Therapist-induced deterioration in psychotherapy. *In* Gurman, A. S. and Razin, A. M. (eds). *Effective Psychotherapy: a Handbook of Research*, 452–81. Oxford: Pergamon Press.

Lazarus, A. (1969). Relationship therapy: often necessary but usually insufficient. *The Counseling Psychologist* 1, 25–7.

Lennard, H. L. and Bernstein, A. (1960). *The Anatomy of Psychotherapy*. New York: Columbia University Press.

Levine, F. M. and Tilker, H. A. (1974). A behaviour modification approach to supervision of psychotherapy. *Psychother.: Theory, Res. and Practice* 11, 182–8.

Matarazzo, R. (1978). Research on the teaching and learning of psycho-therapeutic skills. *In* Garfield, S. L. and Bergin, A. E. (eds). *Handbook of Psychotherapy and Behavior Change*. New York: Wiley.

Mehrabian, A. (1972). *Non-verbal communication*. Chicago: Aldine-Atherton.

Mintz, J., Luborsky, L. and Auerback, A. H. (1971). Dimensions of psycho-therapy: a factor-analytic study of ratings of psychotherapy sessions. *J. Consulting and Clin. Psychol.* 36, 106–20.

Mitchell, K. M., Bozarch, J. D. and Krauft, C. C. (1977). A re-appraisal of the therapeutic effectiveness of accurate empathy, non-possessive warmth and genuineness. *In* Gurman, A. S. and Razin, A. M. (eds). *Effective Psychotherapy: a Handbook of Research*, 482–502. Oxford: Pergamon Press.

Morris, R. J. and Suckerman, K. R. (1974). Therapist warmth as a factor in automated desensitization. *J. Consult. Clin. Psychol.* 42, 244–50.

Parloff, M. B., Waskow, I. E. and Wolfe, B. E. (1978). Research on therapist variables in relation to process and outcome. *In* Garfield, S. L. and Bergin, A. E. (eds). *Handbook of Psychotherapy and Behavior Change*. New York: Wiley.

Patterson, C. H. (1974). *Relationship Counseling and Psychotherapy*. New York: Harper and Row.

Paul, G. L. and McInnis, T. L. (1974). Attitudinal changes associated with two approaches to training mental health technicians in milieu and social learning programs. *J. Consult. Clin. Psychol.* 42, 21–3.

Rogers, C. (1957). The necessary and sufficient conditions of therapeutic personality change. *J. Consult. Psychol.* 21, 95–103.

Rogers, C. (1977). *On Personal Power: Inner Strength and its Revolutionary Impact*. New York: Delacorte Press.

Rice, L. N. (1965). Therapist's style of participation and case outcome. *J. Consult. Psychol.* 29, 155–60.

Rice, L. N. and Wagstaff, A. K. (1967). Client voice quality and expressive style as indexes of productive psychotherapy. *J. Consult. Psychol.* 31, 557–63.

Ricks, D. F. (1974). Supershrink: methods of a therapist judged successful on the basis of adult outcomes of adolescent patients. *In* Ricks, D. F., Roff, M. and Thomas, A. (eds). *Life History Research in Psychopathology*. Minneapolis: University of Minnesota.

Ryan, V. L. and Gizynski, M. N. (1971). Behavior therapy in retrospect: patients' feelings about their behavior therapists. *J. Consult. Clin. Psychol.* 37, 1–9.

Scheflen, A. E. (1965). Quasi-courtship behavior in psychotherapy. *Psychiatry* 28, 245–57.

Seay, T. A. and Altekruse, M. K. (1979). Verbal and non-verbal behavior in judgements of facilitative conditions. *J. Counseling Psychol.* 26, 108–19.

Shapiro, D. A. (1979). Effective psychotherapy: issues, trends and prospects.

In Sutherland, N. S. (ed.). *Tutorial Essays in Psychology, III.* New York: Erlbaum.

Singer, B. A. and Luborky, L. B. (1977). Countertransference: the status of clinical versus quantitative research. *In* Gurman, A. S. and Razin, A. M. (eds). *Effective Psychotherapy: a Handbook of Research*, 433–51. Oxford: Pergamon Press.

Smith, M. L. and Glass, G. V. (1977). Meta-analysis of psychotherapy outcome studies. *Am. Psychol.* 32, 752–60.

Snyder, M. and Monson, T. C. (1975). Persons, situations and the control of social behavior. *J. Personality Soc. Psychol.* 32, 637–44.

Strupp, H. H. (1977). A reformulation of the dynamics of the therapist's contribution. *In* Gurman, A. S. and Razin, A. M. (eds). *Effective Psychotherapy: a Handbook of Research.* Oxford: Pergamon Press.

Strupp, H. H., Hadley, S. W. and Gomes-Schwartz, B. (1977). *Psychotherapy for Better or worse: the Problem of Negative Effects.* New York: Jason-Aronson.

Tourney, G., Bloom, V., Lowinger, P. L., Schorer, G., Auld, F. and Grisell, J. (1966). A study of psychotherapeutic process variables in psychoneurotic and schizophrenic patients. *Am. J. Psychother.* 20, 112–24.

Truax, C. B. and Carkhuff, R. R. (1967). *Toward Effective Counselling and Psychotherapy.* Chicago: Aldine.

Truax, C. B. and Mitchell, K. M. (1971). Research on certain therapist interpersonal skills in relation to process and outcome. *In* Bergin, A. E. and Garfield, S. L. (eds). *Handbook of Psychotherapy and Behavior Change*, 299–344. New York: Wiley.

Vandenbos, G. R. and Karon, B. P. (1971). Pathogenesis: a new therapist personality dimension related to therapeutic effectiveness. *J. Personality Assessment* 35, 252–60.

Weiner, I. (1975). *Principles of Psychotherapy.* New York: Wiley.

Wessler, R. L. and Ellis, A. (1979). Supervision in rational-emotive therapy. *In* Hess, A. R. (ed.). *Psychotherapy Supervision*, 181–91. New York: Wiley.

Wexler, D. A. and Rice, L. N. (eds) (1974). *Innovations in Client-Centred Therapy.* New York: Wiley.

Wills, T. A. (1978). Perceptions of clients by professional helpers. *Psychol. Bull.* 85, 968–1000.

Yalom, I. D. and Lieberman, M. A. (1971). A study of encounter group casualties. *Arch. Gen. Psychiatr.* 25, 16–30.

5 The social casework interview

BARBARA L. HUDSON

Introduction

The range of interpersonal skills relevant to social work is probably greater than for other professions represented in this book, and yet little is known about which skills are necessary or effective. It is tempting to leave the whole question where it has lain for most of social work's short history: buried among imprecise concepts like 'relationship'. 'On the subject of relationship caseworkers are tempted towards rhapsody, mysticism and at times a triumphant vagueness' (Timms 1964, p. 89). But social work teachers have to decide what skills to train even though such decisions lack sound empirical backing. This chapter attempts to tackle the problem in relation to social casework — that is, helping people case by case, rather than in groups or via community organization. It is concerned only with the skills of interpersonal interaction, although there are other essential abilities of at least equal importance. To start with, we can make common-sense deductions about what communication tasks must be performed to achieve particular goals with particular people; and we can refine the resulting syllabus with the help of practice wisdom — the accumulated experience of practitioners as to what seems to work — and the findings of research in our own and related disciplines.

An overview of social work roles and objectives

The task of the social worker is usually defined in very abstract terms. This applies both to his aims and his day-to-day behaviour. Two questions need to be answered: what is a social worker doing when he is 'doing social work', and what is he hoping to achieve? Vagueness on both topics has bedevilled research into social work and the interpretation of findings from what little research has been done. The social worker's goals are as often as not a compromise between the aims of society, the ultimate employer, the immediate employing agency, the profession itself and the client. The compromise can be an uneasy one and sometimes there is conflict between the aims of the worker and of the other party in an interaction; for example, the other party may want to be left alone or to deceive the worker, who for his part seeks to obtain information from the other party or to 'help him change'.

Though counselling is an important part of social work, the skills of the counsellor are not the only skills social workers must develop; and even among those clients for whom some form of counselling may be appropriate, many are not voluntary self-referrals. The British Association of Social Workers (1977) lists twenty roles, of which counselling or therapy is only one. Almost all of these roles include communication with other people. They may be summarized under the headings of 'helping people change', obtaining information, teaching and giving advice, oversight or supervision, and persuading or requesting.

A 'case' may have a variety of desirable outcomes and may require one or many encounters with an interactant, each encounter having within it many moves. During each encounter there may be several intermediate goals, for example in a first meeting with the relative of a psychiatric patient the intermediate goals could be to obtain co-operation, to get information, and to allay feelings of guilt. The moves in this example would include opening the interview, explaining one's role as a helper, sympathetic listening, asking questions, making empathic statements, reassuring and closing the interview. Contacts occur in a variety of settings: the worker's territory or the other person's, or places that belong to neither, a hospital ward, a day centre, a prison cell or a coffee bar. The advantages of casework interviewing while walking or driving are argued by West (1979).

Most casework writing is about the social worker's interaction with an individual in need of help, but this does not do justice to the reality. A distinction must be made between the client system (for whose benefit the work is undertaken), the target system (those whom the worker seeks to influence) and the action system (those whose services are co-ordinated to help the client and change the target)

(Pincus and Minahan 1973). When client and target are the same, the skills of counselling are appropriate; but when the target is not the client we may need different skills: selling an idea, evoking sympathy, making requests effectively. Even controversial tactics may be considered: confrontation, threat, bargaining. Changing the mind of an unsympathetic landlord requires a very different 'front' from comforting a distressed client. It may be hard to persuade the respondent in a fact-finding interview to co-operate. A patient's relative, a landlord or an employer may be articulate, secretive, intimidated or intimidating.

Hence the social worker needs a high level and wide range of general social skills and also more specialized professional ones. He needs to be assertive, rewarding and perceptive – all the qualities that make up everyday social competence. He also has to know the rules of many different social groups. He needs to be able to form a therapeutic relationship and undertake the procedures implicated in the term 'therapy'; he needs the skills of the research interviewer, including those used when the subject matter is intimate or controversial; he needs skills similar to those of the selection interviewer when he is assessing applicants for child-minding or fostering; often his work will resemble that of the doctor seeking to uncover a patient's problem; or when he addresses the court or the large case conference, that of the public speaker.

The foregoing will give some impression of what would be required of a hypothetical caseworker competent in all fields of practice. Specialization by setting (e.g. hospital, prison or school) or by client group (e.g. the mentally ill, the elderly or children) helps to reduce the demand for such a broad array of competencies. But each individual needs a wide repertoire and teachers have to attempt to prepare students for the situations they are most likely to encounter.

Which are the useful skills?

Research evidence

Unfortunately, the social work literature offers few empirically based guidelines. Much of the evaluative research, with its generally disappointing results, has been criticized for using outcome criteria that were not in keeping with the approach of the study social workers. For example, if the researchers' success criterion is fewer delinquent acts, and the workers aim rather for self-awareness and use insight-giving techniques then the researchers' verdict of 'non-effectiveness' becomes questionable: either the goals or the procedures or the performance of the workers, or simply the researchers' criterion, was 'at fault' and we can't know which. Until evaluative research takes this basic problem into consideration not much progress can be made in specifying effective professional behaviour.

An additional drawback is that most research projects have been concerned with broad agency programmes and have not examined the personal attributes or microbehaviours of individual practitioners. At the risk of oversimplifying the studies and their findings, it seems reasonable to conclude from them one very important pointer: traditionally organized training in counselling based on psychodynamic concepts has a poor track record. Qualified social workers have apparently failed to produce change in the behaviour and feelings of certain typical social work clients, such as the delinquent and predelinquent and the poor and the multi-problem family (see Fischer 1973).

One well-designed study throwing some light on the use of counselling procedures by caseworkers is the Casework Methods Project (Reid and Shyne 1969). The clients were voluntary and chiefly middle-class and their problems were of personal/social functioning (but not delinquency, mental illness or addictions). Short-term and time-limited treatment was compared with traditional open-ended treatment; the outcome was significantly better for the experimental group. The caseworkers in the experimental treatment were more 'active' and gave advice more often.

This study has been followed by a proposed model which has received a fair measure of research support (Reid and Epstein 1972). In the first interview the problem is elicited and clarified, goals selected and agreed and tasks formulated. Week by week the worker engages in focusing the discussion, encouraging the client, expressing interest, suggesting further tasks and means to achieve goals. The final interview is spent identifying achievements and discussing how the same approach might be applied to future problems. Here is an apparently successful package, although it is not known which elements are the important ones: time limits, task focus, selection of goals with client agreement, or encouragement for behaviour change outside the interviews. But we are much closer to knowing the kinds of behaviour the worker should learn for work with clients resembling the clients in the study. Until the key ingredients can be identified it would be wise to ensure that students master the total package.

Behavioural casework, which applies behavioural procedures used by other professions (as well as the more specifically social work procedures such as advice and concrete assistance with problems other than personal ones) derives its rationale from the large body of outcome research carried out in psychology and psychiatry. Crisis intervention is another approach which has a great deal of overlap with the work of other professionals. The findings in both fields support those of Reid and his colleagues on time limits, partializing the problem and setting tasks to be performed outside the casework sessions.

Another important study is that by Goldberg (1970). Intervention by qualified and unqualified social workers was compared: the former achieved significantly better outcomes. Here the effective elements are more difficult to unravel. The qualified workers had more time and more supervision; they knew their work was being evaluated; and they used more discrimination in their choice of helping methods and contacted other agencies more often. The two latter points offer important clues regarding effective casework performance.

Other studies have provided information about the kind of worker behaviour that is valued by the people on the receiving end. Hollis (1968) found that drop-out was associated with the use of insight-giving procedures early in the contact. In Mayer and Timms' study (1969), clients who were dissatisfied seem to have had a similar reaction. In this study, working-class clients were interviewed in depth and their views and experiences compared, taking into account whether they had been seeking help with material or interpersonal problems. Dissatisfied clients who had interpersonal problems disliked apparent passivity on the worker's part, focus on the client himself rather than the person he complained about and interest in the client's past rather than his current situation. They took the worker's behaviour to mean that he was not interested, did not understand or was at a loss how to help. The satisfied clients tended to have had workers who seemed less passive, and were supportive–directive rather than reflective or interpretive in approach; these clients received a message of interest and caring and appreciated receiving reassurance and advice. Among those seeking material help the key reason for satisfaction was getting the help they wanted. However, satisfied clients in this group also appreciated being given a chance to discuss other problems and receiving a message of concern and trust in them. Like those with interpersonal problems, the dissatisfied disliked an insight-orientated approach, which some considered nosey or distrustful, and a focus on unhappy personal circumstances, which they found upsetting and pointless. One major difference between satisfied and dissatisfied clients was whether or not they understood what the worker was trying to do. However, Mayer and Timms were unsure as to whether the workers could have 'educated' these clients into accepting the principles underlying their approach.

Sainsbury (1975) obtained similar comments from the mainly satisfied working-class clients of a voluntary agency. They especially valued informality and concrete expressions of concern, and they appreciated advice in such a context. The clients in a Social Services consumer survey (Glampson and Goldberg 1976) also stressed aspects of the relationship. Asked about the qualities of a good social worker they placed greatest emphasis on 'pleasing personality and qualities such as cheerfulness and an ability to take an interest in people' or, in the words of one respondent: 'understanding — a good listener — it's the way they talk to you, make you feel your problem is their problem' (ibid., p. 10). The results of more recent research on clients' attitudes (Aldgate 1977) with working-class parents of children in care agrees with the earlier findings. Once again, 'friendliness' was highly valued, and advice in an atmosphere of friendliness was appreciated. These clients' comments are at variance with the more traditional social work opinion that advice is 'the hallmark of the unskilled in social work' (Bessell 1971, p. 29).

However, these valued-worker behaviours need not necessarily be effective in the sense of achieving the objectives of casework. The findings of the IMPACT series of controlled studies (Folkard, *et al.* 1976) illustrate this point: despite appreciation expressed by most of the probation officers' clients for support and encouragement, and the belief that they had gained in self-awareness, there was no 'impact' on re-conviction rates. Similarly, Sainsbury (1975) reports that changes were most apparent in the area of personal and family feelings — but that these changes in feelings bore no relationship to changes in social functioning. In other words, social casework may be comforting or congenial without leading to behavioural change or to the achievement of concrete, specific objectives.

To summarize the findings of this limited body of research: the most useful and acceptable professional interpersonal skills would appear to be the ability to express caring, to listen responsively and to structure the intervention, specifying objectives and the steps needed to achieve them. 'Talking treatment' should be supplemented by tasks for the client and making use of outside resources. Traditional recommendations to avoid giving advice and to work towards increased self-awareness have received little empirical backing. Since almost all of the studies have focused on the counselling aspect of casework, the many other important activities subsumed under the term 'casework' remain to be studied.

For further empirically based guidelines, we must turn to the work of other disciplines, especially social psychology, and research into activities that social work shares with other professions (see, for example, the reviews of psychotherapy and behavioural therapy literature in Fischer 1978). The reader is also referred to the chapters in this book on psychotherapy (Chapter 4) and on doctor–patient relationships (Chapter 3) and those on selection and research interviewing in its companion volume (Argyle (ed.) 1981). *Social Skills and Work*), as well as the account of 'ordinary' social skills in Chapter 1.

Practice wisdom

The literature of practice wisdom, though often vague and imprecise, contains some helpful guidelines. Much of it parallels the psychotherapy literature. The worker enables the client to express feelings; he reflects back feelings, asks open-ended questions, gives tentative interpretations, uses non-verbal as well as verbal signals to indicate empathy, warmth and genuineness and he is careful to detect clues on the client's state of mind. He seeks to develop a sort of anticipatory empathy, trying to ensure that cultural and role differences between him and his client do not interfere with their communication. He is conscious of the basic asymmetry between his own and the client's position (Fitzjohn 1974), and he analyses his own emotions so as to control their effects on his own communication and his understanding of the client's communication; he also values his own feelings as a source of knowledge about his client. Practice texts discussing these aspects of casework include those by Bessell (1971) and Kadushin (1972).

Social work textbooks give more space than do psychotherapy textbooks to discussion of work with people who are not verbally skilled or who are 'hard to reach' for other reasons. For example, in interviewing the mentally ill, Raven (1974) advises against interpretations and advises caution in permitting ventilation, and stresses the value of stating and restating realities; such advice can be supplemented with some of the practice literature of psychiatry. Another client group singled out in the practice literature is the so-called 'multi-problem' family. It is suggested that workers need to find concrete ways of expressing concern and to recognize openly the feelings of anxiety or anger these clients usually have about 'the Welfare'. Direct work with children is discussed by Holgate (1972) and Berry (1972). Other important differences between client and worker − especially those of culture and language − are emphasized in writing on social work with immigrants (Cheetham 1972, Triseliotis 1972). Awareness of such differences lessens the danger of misunderstanding and being misunderstood. (For detailed discussion of psychological and social influences affecting communication between social workers and those they interview see Day 1977, Cross 1974, Fitzjohn 1974 and Sutton 1979.)

In interactions with persons other than a voluntary client similar skills may come into play. An informant is given the opportunity to express his feelings and these are acknowledged; an attempt is made to help him feel at ease before the business part of the interview begins. Questions about the present come before questions about the past, and neutral topics are discussed before the more intimate ones. The relevance of the questions to the aims of the interview is explained. However, behaviour appropriate to a counselling interview must not become over-generalized. I have had the experience of being the 'interviewee' of a social worker who consistently reflected back, empathized and seemed to be trying to elicit feelings, when I was seeking information, not therapy. Relatives of psychiatric patients − ostensibly providing information for the psychiatrist − have complained of the incomprehensible approach of social workers interviewing them.

Types of social work interaction other than the warm, sympathetic style are rarely discussed in the literature. A notable exception is Pincus and Minahan's book (1973). Besides the more desirable collaborative relationships there are also bargaining ones, when the worker offers some advantage to the other person in return for co-operation; and conflictual ones, where the worker seeks to coerce others to achieve benefit for his client. The chapter on 'Exercising

Influence' considers these kinds of relationship in some detail (ibid., pp. 247–71). Inducement is one form of exercising influence: using rewards or sanctions to obtain co-operation. Clearly there are major ethical questions to be considered, although in much direct work with clients milder versions of the same thing are common; benefit, usually in the form of social reinforcement, is often made contingent upon the client's co-operation. One of the few texts other than Pincus and Minahan's to discuss in detail both the skills of 'assertive' casework and the characteristics of clients for whom these techniques may be appropriate is that by Foren and Bailey (1968). The skills required resemble those taught in assertiveness training programmes (Sundel and Sundel 1980). Social workers seem to find such skills particularly difficult to exercise, perhaps because of commitment to client self-determination and unconditional acceptance: two cornerstones of social work's value system. Persuasion is another means of influence discussed by Pincus and Minahan. The worker needs to be able to assemble appropriate information and to present it clearly and forcefully. He needs to appear authoritative as well as attractive and caring.

Behavioural social work writers give more specific guidelines for action. For example, Schwartz and Goldiamond (1975) provide an interview format almost word for word. Social workers using this approach may attempt to extinguish anxiety by presenting a hierarchy to clients trained in relaxation, or encouraging talk about anxiety-provoking topics while themselves remaining calm and supportive. They give verbal reinforcement accompanied by non-verbal signs of interest and concern when the client has performed or reported certain adaptive behaviours. They may look away, interrupt, change the subject or state their disapproval in response to unproductive or pessimistic talk. They may talk about themselves or demonstrate desired behaviours. They may systematically teach such activities as decision making or playing with a child. Unlike more traditional caseworkers, they regularly give advice and directions. However, the skills of the behavioural social worker will always include those of the non-behaviourist, such as the expression of empathy and warmth.

Assembling a practice-skills curriculum

The social work teacher faced with such an array of possible syllabus components often allows the students' immediate concerns and current fieldwork needs to dictate the teaching content. For systematic training a repertoire of skills for commonly met situations must be selected and subdivided (unscrambled) into elements that can be observed and taught. This can be attempted in the following ways.

By setting

For example, the probation officer in court. He needs to follow court etiquette, to speak briefly, coherently and fluently and to give NV signs of confidence without disrespect. He needs to be understandable and believable, and must command respect.

By roles

For example, the social worker visiting a foster home. He is part-supervisor, part-colleague, and at times part-therapist. He needs ordinary conversational skills, keen powers of observation and an ability to keep the discussion focused on the professional business of the interchange.

By characteristics of the interactant

For example, the aggressive or paranoid client. The worker has to focus the interview to indicate understanding and respect without either confirming or arguing about the other's delusions. He needs to be able to calm the client, perhaps distract him from a delusional train of thought on to a shared reality. His own anxiety must not be allowed to become translated into behaviours such as might be mistaken for anger or suspicion.

By stage in the case

At the beginning the worker has to explain his own role and the expectations he has of the other's role. He needs to give an impression of good will, competence and confidence. Again, feelings of uncertainty or anxiety must not be communicated. Clients who are overanxious need to be reassured and given a message of hope; those who are not anxious enough – the 'unmotivated' – may need to be encouraged towards a realistic response to their situation.

By stage of the interview

For example, at the beginning the client is given a chance to settle in before the business part of the meeting. The interview is closed sufficiently gradually so that the other person does not feel he is being brusquely dismissed, and yet sufficiently firmly so that he recognizes that the meeting is over.

By 'move'

For example: making an interpretation in a questioning, gentle tone; confronting the client with an unpleasant reality in unequivocal language and firm but not unfriendly manner; giving social reinforcement with attention to its NV aspects in a manner that to this individual does not seem either lukewarm or gushing.

The document *Learning to be a Probation Officer* (Central Council for Training and Education in Social Work 1978) selects key situations by legal status (prisoner, juvenile under supervision); by characteristics (depressed, manipulative, passive); by setting (office, court, prison, home); and by role of interactant (other professional, client, volunteer). Others focus on more specific skills or moves: questioning, explaining, reinforcement, sustaining, reflecting back feelings and paraphrasing (Hargie, *et al.* 1978). Some descriptions give less detail; for example Howard and Gooderham (1975) select as 'main issues' NV communication, meaningful response to client needs, observation, the feeling content of the interview and the worker's self-awareness. Most courses emphasize the key counselling qualities of empathy, warmth and genuineness (Fischer 1978, Thomas, *et al.*, unpublished document). The latter group grade their practice sessions according to difficulty, beginning with the voluntary client who comes to the office, and moving to interviews with non-voluntary clients, more than one interactant and different settings. They also select beginning an interview, asking questions, dealing with silences and making contracts. On our own course we have chosen to focus on the therapeutic qualities of empathy, warmth and genuineness, plus the minutiae of interview skills: picking up NV cues and signals, questioning, attending behaviours and the like. Next we address more difficult tasks: asking embarrassing questions, introducing upsetting topics, refusing requests, confronting and focusing an interview with an aggressive or domineering interactant.

In later sessions the students practise explaining their role to a variety of audiences, including clients, informants and other workers.

None of these syllabuses has backing other than teachers' beliefs about what is relevant and important for beginning social workers. The most systematic attempt to identify and specify key situations which social workers must be capable of handling, and what are the most effective responses in those situations, is by Rose, *et al.* (1977). A set of six scenes was developed from suggestions by social work practitioners rated for relevance and difficulty. These scenes included dealing with the uncooperative client and informing a client that material aid will not be forthcoming. Examples of worker behaviour in the situations were rated in terms of identifying the client's feelings, expressing feeling on the worker's part, expressing opinions, persistence (maintaining one's point of view in the face of increasing demands), giving clarification, seeking clarification, timing, appropriate affect, latency, voice level and fluency. These categories were further itemized: for example, under 'expressing feelings' — the use of 'I' statements — and under 'clarification' — the suggestion of worker and client working jointly on a problem. Rose and his colleagues comment that the six situations and the associated skills, which are used in role-play tests of interpersonal competence, may not be representative of the wide range of problematic situations that social workers encounter; and research in the field is continuing. There is some similarity between the areas identified in this study and those taught in programmes described earlier: for example, in the author's department therapeutic skills and the assertive skills of confrontation and refusing requests are among the areas focused on. Our selection has received positive feedback from students who mention the frequency with which they encountered situations in which the skills chosen were needed in the field. However, many more items are suggested for inclusion in the syllabus than can be covered in the time available.

The teaching of practice skills

Having selected the skills to train, what teaching programmes should be constructed for the purpose? First, it might be useful to review current training arrangements.

Traditional training arrangements

Academic study   In educational establishments most of the teaching time is occupied with acquiring knowledge that is supposed to inform the worker's selection of goals and methods and his understanding of the people he seeks to help and the systems that affect them. Much of this content can be related to attitudes towards people and to the making of intervention plans in broad outline: it forms an essential background to the learning of practice skills. Besides the contributory disciplines of sociology, psychology and social policy, casework approaches or models are studied and discussed. However, exposure to this varied material can present problems in translating knowledge into action. As Sheldon (1978) has argued, the implications of theories presented as equally valid may be mutually incompatible, and the student seeking to relate both psychodynamic theory and learning theory to practice (to take a particularly difficult example) may find himself unable to construct a logical, coherent intervention plan. Besides, Fischer (1978) points out that most of the literature from the contributory disciplines and also much of the casework writing deals with explanation and assessment with little reference to the skills of intervention − and understanding a problem is not the same as helping to solve it.

Fieldwork supervision   About 50 per cent of course time is spent in social work agencies and it is here that the linking of theory and practice and the development of practice skills is expected to take place. The student provides written records of his activities and discusses his work in supervision sessions. The supervisor gives feedback and advice on future action and seeks to guide the student in understanding the problem and his own part in interactions with clients and others. The emphasis is on thinking about the case and speculating about the meaning of each person's behaviour and the feelings of both parties and their origins. The advantages of this type of 'apprenticeship' training include the opportunity to apply theory to practice in the real world. The student can discover practical instances to illustrate, confirm or refute hypotheses derived from the theoretical content of the course; conversely, he can begin to build new hypotheses from his observations. The system allows the student time and advice in planning the content of his work. The emphasis on inner states helps in interpreting the behaviour of others, making accurate empathy more probable, and in dealing more effectively with feelings on the student's part that might interfere with his performance.

However, this system has several drawbacks. It has been criticized by Rothman (1977) who comments that 'the social work profession may no longer be viewed as an apprentice trade', and by Lewis and Gibson (1977) who conclude on the basis of their skills-laboratory experience that traditional fieldwork teaching is inadequate for the development of practice competence. Perhaps the most serious drawback is that a large proportion of the learning is by trial and error; this might have implications for the standard of service received by clients, and it is a slow and inefficient — if at times vivid and unforgettable — way of learning.

Since the student is given responsibility for a case load of his own, the grading of tasks from the less to the more difficult is not feasible, nor is the partializing of skills to be mastered. Then there is the problem of the inadequate data available to the supervisor, who has to rely on the student's recollection of events that may have occurred several days before their discussion. An early study of the use of a tape-recorder as compared with written 'process' records of casework interviews (Itzin 1960) found that more than half of the observations regarded as significant were not included in the written records. Burian (1976) also stresses that the system does not allow the opportunity to try out a better approach immediately. Lastly, although there are spin-offs for the 'doing' from the attention given to the thinking and feeling components of casework, the student's overt behaviour does seem a somewhat neglected facet of total performance. There is a four-link chain: covert behaviours of worker (thoughts, feelings, attitudes) → overt behaviours of worker → covert behaviours of the other person → overt behaviours of the other. The link that gets least attention is the overt behaviours of the worker. Yet worker activity is the part that could, in theory, be most accurately observed, taught and evaluated. The hypothesized inner states are certainly important but are considerably harder to be clear about. The focus on inner states at the expense of overt behaviour seems to be due not only to the circumstances of supervision but also the influence of psychodynamic theory on casework practice.

Learning by observation   Only rarely does a student observe a more experienced worker. It is a curious fact about social work that many of its practitioners have never been seen in action by their colleagues. In certain specialist settings they see another professional — perhaps a psychiatrist on a ward round or a co-therapist in marital therapy.

Whether these are appropriate models for social workers is hard to determine.

Experiential groups These are common in social work training. A stated aim of such groups is the development of awareness of one's own and others' feelings, and of how one's behaviour affects others. The leaders are group therapists of varied theoretical background who are rarely members of the social work profession. One possible consequence of this may be the observation of inappropriate models for practice: there is no evidence on this count. Nor indeed has the proposition that the group experience improves practice been subject to systematic evaluation. One study assessed the effects on the social workers themselves, as measured by changes in neuroticism scores and the opinions of relatives or close friends. The participants had higher neuroticism scores after the group but the informants rated them as more open and more sensitive to others. The researcher suggests that the test scores reflected not a true increase in neuroticism, but rather a greater self-awareness and openness (Cooper 1974). This conclusion, if correct, taken together with other findings on the effect of such groups on non-patient populations (see Gibb 1971), is encouraging as far as it goes. But others have suggested that there is cause for caution. Several studies (Lieberman, *et al.* 1973, Hartley, *et al.* 1976, Galinsky and Schopler 1977) indicate that 'groups may be dangerous'. Further, a controlled study by Brook (1978) produced very mixed results for social work students receiving sensitivity-group training. The experimental group showed a decrease in self-ratings in relationship skills and in self-concept while the control students gained in these measures; and relationship skills as rated by fieldwork teachers were not enhanced by the group experience (except for 'authenticity'). Yet the participants themselves contradicted the experimental findings, claiming that the sensitivity group had improved their self-confidence and skill, and felt strongly that such groups are relevant and useful in social work training. It seems reasonable to suppose that if greater sensitivity and self-awareness and more satisfactory interpersonal skills do result, then these gains might generalize to professional situations. However, the matter is by no means settled. Also, the positive findings are for Rogerian and group analytic groups. The effects on social work students of the Bion-style groups which are often provided have not been studied, and one study of patients' experience of such groups (Malan, *et al.* 1976) produced negative results.

Role play This is occasionally used in social work training. Often it is used as trigger material for case discussions and for sensitizing students to the feelings aroused both in workers and clients. Its value when used in this way has not been assessed. There is, however, one study of the effects of a single experience of role play with video feedback (Star 1977). The dependent variable was students' self-image, measured on a semantic differential. There were definite effects, but these eventually dissipated. Also, the direction of the effect on individual students was towards greater *or* lesser self-confidence, and whether these changes related to the student's true level of skill was not examined. In this, as in other instances, self-awareness is the main aim and whether such experiences improve performance at work remains to be tested.

Most of these approaches reflect the profession's emphasis on self-awareness and on empathy in the sense of feeling what the other may be feeling rather than skill in *communicating* empathy. Progress in skills training requires operational definitions of empathy and other key interpersonal behaviours, in order to label them for the learner, demonstrate them and give practice in them.

Recent developments in training

Schemes that successfully apply these operational definitions are being developed in several educational establishments, and more sophisticated training methods are coming into use. One such scheme is described by Strutt (1974). The scheme included 15 minutes' role-play of work situations and 'live' interviews of other students, with either detailed written scripts or oral instructions on the scene to be enacted, as well as directions about appropriate skills. Each student acted as interviewer and interviewee on two occasions, and video and verbal feedback was given. Two of the findings are of particular interest: the directive trainer was judged more helpful than the non-directive trainer; and at follow-up one year later 85 per cent of the participants believed that they had benefited from the training. Howard and Gooderham (1975) describe a similar brief programme with ten-minute interviews after which various issues were brought out in discussion.

A more systematic scheme is that of Hargie, Tittmar and Dickson (1978), whose paper is to date the most useful British account of a programme of this kind for social workers. The key elements of their training are labelling and analysing the skills to be practised and giving the rationale behind them; role play lasting ten minutes per person (including tutors), giving practice in each skill area (the skills selected are mentioned on p. 119); video feedback; feedback from the person who played the client; and feedback from the rest of the group.

Fischer (1978) describes the training programme for learning the 'core conditions' (empathy, warmth and genuineness) developed for social work students at the University of Hawaii. This programme has been evaluated by rating levels of communication of the core conditions before and after each course. Since it is rare to find detailed proposals for a skills training scheme and even rarer to find a scheme whose effectiveness has been empirically examined, Fischer's model deserves very serious consideration. It is derived from the work of authors teaching the core conditions to a variety of professional groups (for example, Carkhuff 1971) and the microcounselling approach of Ivey (1971). The key principles are as follows: a focus on the scales assessing empathy, warmth and genuineness; intellectual understanding of the rationale for this focus; emphasis on perform-ance as well as discussion; modelling by the instructor; graduated learning experiences; feedback; enjoyable experiences; helping students develop their own style; dual emphasis on client self-exploration and action; range of experience for learners; and evaluation of the results of training (ibid., pp. 325–30). Fischer gives specific directions on how to organize the class, describes the exercises, use of tapes and so on. Intensive role play with videotape feedback in an atmosphere of informality is the central component of this programme.

The phases of the course are set out in detail (ibid., pp. 330–43). The practical part of the programme begins with each student recording an interview for play-back later in the course. They listen to tapes by experienced counsellors and read interview transcripts to obtain experience of a variety of models and to practise identifying the core conditions. Next there are a series of warm-up and intro-ductory exercises or 'games'. This initial phase concludes with teaching about the total casework model proposed by Fischer and its central skill components: attending, responding, exploring and initiating action.

The second phase focuses step by step on attending behaviour, 'body language', accurate listening, expressing and detecting feelings, helping clients speak about problems and voice training. In the third phase the tapes made at the start of the course are rated and discussed; there is further experience of filmed models, further training in expressing the core conditions, and in putting these skills together. Phase four continues the process of discriminating and expressing empathy, warmth and genuineness, practice in 'concreteness' (referring specifically to this client rather than people in general, and encouraging the client to do likewise), focusing on the present, use of self-disclosure and confrontation (the clarification of discrepancies in the client's communications). Towards the end the students are shown tapes made earlier to demonstrate the progress that they have achieved, interviews with real clients are recorded and analysed, and students continue the programme on an informal basis, reviewing their work throughout the field placement. They are encouraged to continue this after they have qualified.

It will be seen that Fischer (1978) and Hargie, Tittmar and Dickson (1978) have included most of the training procedures which will now be suggested on the basis of the literature on learning. They are essentially the same as those used in skills training for other professionals and client groups.

(1) Labelling (identifying) the components to be learned, and giving a theoretical rationale for them. This makes generalization to new situations more probable.

(2) Modelling. Models can be filmed or live. The most effective models have certain qualities: reward success, similarity to the observer. There is evidence in favour of multiple models. This suggests that teachers and fellow students may be appropriate models. Both the specific labelling and the modelling overcome the problems for students caused by their teachers' predilection for vague concepts such as 'giving insight', 'avoiding countertransference', 'confronting'.

(3) Practice. The value of modelling is enhanced if immediate practice is given.

(4) The value of practice is enhanced if feedback is given. Feedback can be received covertly — by viewing oneself in action — or overtly in comments from others, including the person on the receiving end. Reinforcement is combined with feedback. The literature on shaping suggests that reinforcement should be positive, and should be given for successive approximations to the

desired end performance. A group that is supportive can provide this kind of experience, and if this is combined with video feed-back and the opportunity of repeated practice then the optimal conditions for skills improvement will have been met.

(5) Optimal levels of motivation and anxiety. Again, the group culture − which will owe much to the tutor in charge − is of key importance, to ensure that students are sufficiently motivated and, what is more usually an issue, are not so anxious that their performance is disrupted. This is particularly important, since some disruption in skilled performance may be expected when its components are unscrambled for microtraining.

Problems and solutions in skill training on a social work course

Training that includes all the components listed above is a time-consuming business and is possibly problematic in other respects. There are no completely satisfactory solutions but a few tentative suggestions can be made.

Time requirements　In my experience lack of space in an already overcrowded timetable is a major stumbling block. Fischer's (1978) programme takes up to sixty hours (four hours per week over fifteen weeks), and even so might be criticized for teaching only *some* of the necessary skills (those of counselling). This is more than the whole time allotted to casework teaching on many courses. Only one con-structive proposal seems feasible: that more practice teaching should be transferred from the field to the academic establishment (Rothman 1977).

To avoid wasting time on skills the students already possess it is useful to check on ordinary interaction and interview skills first, beginning with a relatively stress-free, brief interview. After this only some of the more problematic microbehaviours will require additional work − perhaps, for one student, NV components; for another use of vocabulary may be the area that needs shaping up. And there is much to be said for grouping students according to special interests, so that after training in the more general skills each group can move on to more specialized ones. For example, those interested in psychiatric work could practise interviewing psychotic patients and explaining their role to other psychiatric staff; others could practise communicating with children, talking with foster parents and interviewing prospective adopters.

Time can be saved by limiting the amount of general discussion before role play and by preparing vignettes to give to role players. Scenes are best kept brief — not longer than fifteen minutes. I am grateful to Robert Liberman for teaching me the time-saving (and assertive) leader behaviour of nominating role players swiftly and in a manner that discourages the shy refusal or the lengthy discussion that a request for volunteers so often brings in its train.

Objections to use of role play and video   Some role-play partners are very convincing and the experience of role reversal provides the possibility of improving one's empathy with the feelings of the person portrayed. However, it is sometimes argued that role plays are not realistic, because of lack of acting ability or life experience or, occasionally, out of rancour — for example, by playing an exceptionally hostile consultant psychiatrist or headmaster (examples from Sheldon 1979). Sheldon attempted two solutions. The first was to bring carefully chosen and prepared clients to the class. This did not prove helpful: the clients couldn't act either, and the students behaved more tentatively towards them than they apparently would in normal circumstances. The second solution was to use drama students. This proved very successful, and the effort to recruit such role partners seems worth pursuing. Another related objection is that the student's enactment of a caseworker in class is different from his 'real' performance in the field. This view is contradicted by Fischer (1978) who states that 'over several years of ratings, no consistent differences between ratings of role-played and actual interviews by the same person have emerged' (p. 331.).

Anxiety or embarrassment   The key to helping students feel comfortable with this form of training lies in the creation of a cohesive and accepting group. Thomas, *et al.* (unpublished document) recommend that numbers should be no more than six. Fischer (1978) stresses informal relationships, leader modelling of warmth and positive responses, jokes and warm-up games. Allowing students to become familiar with the equipment and with being filmed before training proper begins is also helpful. Sheldon (1979) begins with films of *faux pas* by previous students and by staff to reassure the students and create a light-hearted atmosphere. I show an excessively bad performance and then an 'acceptable' but not perfect one. Staff willingness to participate seems a very important ingredient in the initial stages.

Equipment While video offers major advantages – providing instant and comprehensive feedback, and facilitating accurate pin-pointing and modelling of behaviour – there is no evidence that it is essential. Audiotape-recorders are used by some courses, as indeed they were used in the original studies of core therapy conditions and the training courses focusing on them. Day (1977) stresses the value of tape-recording over written process records. If neither is available, programmes such as Fischer's (1978) or Liberman's Personal Effectiveness training (Liberman, *et al.* 1975) can be usefully adapted for social work students. Besides role play, several 'games' can be used to draw attention to and give rapid practice in microbehaviours. Such games include: saying numbers accompanied by NV signs to indicate various emotional states; asking open-ended questions round the circle; miming different moods; recounting a sad or happy experience to a partner who reports or reflects back, and then receives feedback on his level of empathy; no doubt the reader can devise others. Besides being time-saving ways of learning, such games can act as 'warm-ups' for the teaching sessions. Having students perform very short sequences and games lessens the risk of inaccurate recall of the longer role play.

The sort of training I have described is never 'enough'. One hopes that students can transfer their skill and confidence in role play and their ability to analyse the components of a performance to new situations so that they will be able to prepare, with their supervisors' help, for problematic encounters. In fieldwork supervision the re-enactment of an interview will greatly help the supervisor to help the student. Training in new skills and monitoring of those already learned should continue in fieldwork and indeed after qualification. Access to equipment and assistance in the use of these training procedures should ideally be available to agency supervisors as well as course tutors.

Concluding remarks

Any teaching programme has to be tentative and provisional; but what little knowledge there is about social work skills and how to learn them could be used to better effect. Certain trends in social work today seem to be assisting this development. Efforts are being made to define the goals and tasks of casework in ways that are translatable into observable behaviours. Newer casework approaches − task-centred and behavioural − require the specification of input and goals. Psychologists are taking over the teaching on human growth and behaviour from psychoanalysts, and their influence also leads in this direction. In some fields of practice, notably adult psychiatry and probation, social workers are learning to teach social skills to people who are deficient in them; the methods they use and the demands this treatment approach makes in terms of analysing skilled performance and rehearsing its components have an indirect but powerful influence on the profession's own training arrangements.

Professional education involves acquiring theoretical knowledge and practical skills. The expansion of the former in recent years has been considerable; perhaps skills acquisition will soon follow suit. However, I shall end on a note of caution. Technical expertise (know-how) must not be stressed at the expense of know-what and why. The professional must be capable of starting with one plan and adapting or abandoning it in response to changing circumstances; and skilled performance must be used in the furtherance of an intervention plan that promises to be effective. It is ethically unacceptable to consider process without reference to its outcome. A depressing reminder of how far we still have to go was given to me by a psychiatrist who likened the 'socially skilled social worker' to a restaurant where you are made to feel comfortable and valued − but there isn't any food! Growing demands for a proper accounting of the costs and benefits of what social workers do may eventually lead to a better understanding of what 'works' in social work.

References

Aldgate, J. (1977). *Identification of Factors Influencing Children's Length of Stay in Care*. Ph.D. Thesis, University of Edinburgh.

Berry, J. (1972). *Social Work with Children*. London: Routledge and Kegan Paul.

Bessell, R. (1971). *Interviewing and Counselling*. London: Batsford.

British Association of Social Workers (1977). *The Social Work Task*. Birmingham: British Association of Social Workers.

Brook, B. D. (1978). Sensitivity training in social work education. *Br. J. Soc. Work* 8, 193−6.

Burian, W. A. (1976). The laboratory as an element in social work curriculum design. *J. Educ. Soc. Work* 12, 1.

Carkhuff, R. R. (1971). *The Development of Human Resources*. New York: Holt, Rinehart and Wilson.

Central Council for Education and Training in Social Work (1978). *Paper 18: Learning to be a Probation Officer*. London: Central Council for Education and Training in Social Work.

Cheetham, J. (1972). *Social Work with Immigrants*. London: Routledge and Kegan Paul.

Cooper, C. L. (1974). Psychological disturbance following T-groups; relationship between the Eysenck Personality Inventory and family/friends' perceptions. *Br. J. Soc. Work* 4, 39—49.

Cross, C. P. (ed.) (1974). *Interviewing and Communication in Social Work*. London: Routledge and Kegan Paul.

Day, P. R. (1977). *Methods of Learning Communication Skills*. Oxford: Pergamon Press.

Fischer, J. (1973). Is casework effective? A review. *Soc. Work* 18, 107—10.

——— (1978). *Effective Casework Practice: an Eclectic Approach*. New York: McGraw-Hill.

Fitzjohn, J. (1974). An interactionist view of the social work interview. *Br. J. Soc. Work* 4, 425—33.

Folkard, N. S., Smith, D. E. and Smith, D. D. (1976). *IMPACT. Home Office Research Studies*. London: HMSO, vol. 2.

Foren, R. and Bailey, R. (1968). *Authority in Social Casework*. Oxford: Pergamon Press.

Galinsky, M. J. and Schopler, J. H. (1977). Warning: Groups may be dangerous. *Soc. Work* 22, 89—94.

Gibb, J. R. (1971). The effects of human relations training. *In* Bergin, A. E. and Garfield, J. L. (eds). *Handbook of Psychotherapy and Behaviour Change*. New York: Wiley.

Glampson, A. and Goldberg, E. (1976). Post-Seebohm social services (2). *Soc. Work Today* 8, 7—12.

Goldberg, E. M. (1970). *Helping the Aged*. London: Allen and Unwin.

Hargie, O., Tittmar, H. and Dickson, D. (1978). Micro-training: a systematic approach to social work practice. *Soc. Work Today* 9, 14—16.

Hartley, D., Roback, H. B. and Abramowitz, S. I. (1976). Deterioration effects in encounter groups. *Am. Psychol.* 31, 247—55.

Holgate, E. (1972). *Communicating with Children*. London: Longman.

Hollis, F. (1968). Continuance and discontinuance in marital counselling and some observations on joint interviews. *Soc. Casework* 49, 167—74.

Howard, J. and Gooderham, P. (1975). Closed circuit TV in social work training. *Soc. Work Today* 6, 194—7.

Itzin, F. (1960). The use of tape recording in fieldwork. *Soc. Casework* 41, 4.

Ivey, A. E. (1971). *Microcounselling: Innovations in interview training*. Springfield, Ill.: Charles C. Thomas.

Kadushin, A. (1972). *The Social Work Interview*. New York: Columbia.

Lewis, J. and Gibson, F. (1977). The teaching of some social work skills: Towards a skills laboratory. *Br. J. Soc. Work* 3, 189—210.

Liberman, R. P., King, L. W., De Risi, W. J. and McCann, M. (1975). *Personal Effectiveness*. Champaign, Illinois: Research Press.

Lieberman, M. A., Yalom, I. D. and Miles, M. B. (1973). *Encounter Groups: First Facts*. New York: Basic Books.

Malan, P. M., Balfour, F. M., Hood, V. G. and Shooter, A. M. (1976). Group psychotherapy: a long term follow-up study. *Arch. Gen. Psychiatr.* 33, 1305–15.

Mayer, J. E. and Timms, N. (1969). *The Client Speaks: Working Class Impressions of Casework*. London: Routledge and Kegan Paul.

Pincus, A. and Minahan, A. (1973). *Social Work Practice: Model and Method*. Itasca, Ill.: F. E. Peacock.

Raven, S. (1974). Interviewing in special situations. *In* Cross, C. P. (ed.). *Interviewing and Communication in Social Work*. London: Routledge and Kegan Paul.

Reid, W. and Shyne, A. (1969). *Brief and Extended Casework*. New York: Columbia.

Reid, W. and Epstein, L. (1972). *Task Centred Casework*. New York: Columbia University Press.

Rose, S. D., Cayner, J. J. and Edleson, J. L. (1977). Measuring interpersonal competence. *Soc. Work* 22, 125–40.

Rothman, J. (1977). Development of a profession: Field instruction correlates. *Soc. Service Rev.* 51, 289–310.

Sainsbury, E. (1975). *Social Work with Families*. London: Routledge and Kegan Paul.

Schwartz, A. and Goldiamond, I. (1975). *Social Casework: A Behavioral Approach*. New York: Columbia University Press.

Sheldon, B. (1978). Theory and practice in social work: A re-examination of a tenuous relationship. *Br. J. Soc. Work* 8, 1.

———— (1979). Putting realism into rehearsed simulations. *Soc. Work Today*. 11, 11–14.

Star, B. (1977). The effects of videotape self-image confrontation on helping perceptions. *J. Educ. Soc. Work* 13, 1–6.

Strutt, B. (1974). Role play: a training technique. *In* Cross, C. P. (ed.). *Interviewing and Communication in Social Work*. London: Routledge and Kegan Paul.

Sundel, M. and Sundel, S. S. (1980). *Be Assertive: A Practical Guide for Human Service Workers*. New York: Sage Publications.

Sutton, C. (1979). *Psychology for Social Workers and Counsellors*. London: Routledge and Kegan Paul.

Timms, N. (1964). *Social Casework: Principles and Practice*. London: Routledge and Kegan Paul.

Triseliotis, J. (ed.) (1972). *Social Work with Coloured Immigrants and Their Families*. Oxford University Press.

West, D. (1979). The social casework interview. *Soc. Work Today* 10, 20–1.

6 A social skills approach to childrearing

MYRNA SHURE

Introduction

This chapter focuses on children's development of social skills and the influence of childrearing practices upon this development.

Based on discoveries of researchers and therapists, strategies and techniques have been applied to systematic childrearing training programmes to help parents foster optimal social adjustment and interpersonal competence in their children. These programmes can be viewed as following a sequence from changing the parents' attitudes and behaviour towards their children to training parents how to include the child as a participant in the process and training the child in specific skills via the parent. The first two types of programmes (referred to as parent-focused training) emphasize modifying parents, the implications being that children would favourably respond to that change. The remaining type of programme (referred to as child-focused training) stresses parents' helping their children to learn specific social skills of their own.

In my view, social skills go beyond how people *act*. In relating to others these skills also include how people think, because in the interpersonal world how they think affects what they do. When, for example, a 4-year-old tried to grab a toy from his friend, could he also think of other ways to get the toy? Did he think of potential consequences of grabbing and if so, would he have chosen a different option (if he could think of one)? As specific thinking skills associated with healthy social development are identified, how parents can and do contribute to these skills is learned. This chapter will also address how key thought processes vary at different ages, and their application to and implications for a social skills approach to child-rearing.

Parent-focused training

As research investigating childrearing practices which are associated with healthy social development in children became known, it also became clear that effective techniques were more typically applied by parents in the middle than in the lower socioeconomic classes. With this in mind, some researchers, educators and mental health practitioners began to focus their efforts on the poor, built on the premise that if parents could learn these techniques then the chances for optimum social development of their children would increase. Given cost-effectiveness, availability of government funds and primary prevention as a research and service goal, emphasis began to shift from traditional individual child or family service therapy to an educational model of group parent training.

The advent of educational programmes to enhance social skills is important, because throughout the 1960s and early 1970s most group educational parent training programmes focused on advancing verbal and intellectual skills in lower-class children — the goal being to improve the likelihood of later school achievement (see Parker 1972). While such cognitive skills may be an integral part of a child's total development, researchers such as Bronfennbrenner (1974) stated the need to promote positive mental health, and those such as Schaefer (1977) added the need to focus on the positive, not the negative, and to identify strengths, skills, competence and adjustment, not just symptoms, deficiencies and deviant behaviour.

Although group parent training programmes designed to enhance social skills and development are still relatively few in number, the work of Sears, *et al.* (1957), Becker (1964) and Hoffman (1970*b*) have had a large effect on the techniques and goals of some of them. Johnson, *et al.* (1976) began training Mexican–American parents when their children were a year old and helped parents learn to show their children affection, to apply non-restrictive but firm control and to encourage verbal interaction, particularly reasoning and explanation for instructions, commands and discipline. These attitudes and strategies were fostered because the above-mentioned research on which their programmes was based showed them to be associated with healthy impulse control and mature moral development. In contrast, physical punishment and verbal coercion, techniques likely to be applied more often by parents in the lower classes, were commonly linked with frustration, anger and aggression.

Whereas children in the study by Johnson, *et al.* are too young to evaluate the effects of their programme on interpersonal skill development, Wittes and Radin (1969*c*) have applied another finding of Sears, *et al.* (1957) to their training — that impulse control is achieved when the warm relationship with a parent is contingent upon good behaviour. Because their complete curriculum for parents included various other techniques and goals (Wittes and Radin 1969*a*, *b*) and because their research goal was to compare teaching techniques (lecture with discussion) (Wittes and Radin 1971, Radin 1972), they did not intend to evaluate the specific effect of applying reinforcement techniques to enhance social skill development. However, Combs and Slaby (1979) present evidence that reinforcement techniques alone do not generally last beyond the period of training. Once reinforcement ceases the desired behaviours may well decrease, because the children have not learned to think about what they do but rather have acquired behaviour patterns from association with immediate reward and punishment.

Recognizing that the prime focus of pure behaviour modification techniques is to shape behaviours through association with reward and punishment (see Mahoney 1974, Meichenbaum 1977), Slaby (unpublished observations) helped parents of disturbed nursery children to learn to communicate their expectations clearly — particularly by emphasizing to the child what to do, not primarily what not to do. Mothers (and teachers) were taught to suggest appropriate alternatives when children would do something unacceptable, such as 'You can ask for that' (when they grab a toy); 'Tell him, "I'm playing with this" ' (when a child grabs a toy from him); or 'Tell him "no hitting" ' or 'turn away' (when the child is hit). Based on Hoffman's (1970*a*) report that induction strengthens mature moral development, Slaby also encouraged parents to explain the effect of their behaviour on others. In his earlier work with 4-year-olds, Hoffman (1963) found that children who showed the most consideration for others had mothers who focused attention on the motives and feelings of others, through such statements as 'You hurt his feelings'. Hoffman and Saltzstein (1967) add that when consequences are explained the effect of children's behaviour on others is focused, which theoretically should inhibit them from hurting others, or their feelings.

Amount and quality of parent communication is crucial in any family, and the lack of it is particularly evident in parents whose youngsters already display severe behaviour problems. Heinicke (1976, 1977) found that mothers of disturbed nursery children became more available, more communicative and more affectionate when helped to understand and articulate their own problems, as well as those they experienced in childrearing. Their children's school behaviour and peer relations consequently improved significantly. Baldwin and Baldwin (1976 and personal communication) found that similar counselling techniques decreased the amount of coercion imposed, increased the positive affect shown, and enhanced the quality and frequency of parent–child interaction. As Cole (unpublished observations) points out, however, too many *and* too few behaviour requests, suggestions to help and requests for information can damagingly influence a child's social competence.

Thus it seems that how parents talk to their children, how often they do so and the degree of warmth and affection they feel and communicate all play a critical role in the child's developing social behaviour and competence.

But there is more. Baumrind (1967) has found that parents who not only communicate clearly what is expected of their children when demands or requests are made but who also encourage their children to express their own feelings and opinions have more socially competent children than those who do not. This implies a different childrearing style; that of encouraging children to engage in the process of solving typical, everyday problems that come up with peers and figures of authority.

One parent training programme that engages the child in the problem solving process is Thomas Gordon's well-established Parent Effectiveness Training, also known as PET. Because of the widespread popularity of this programme in the USA (over 250 000 parents have been trained in workshops [Gordon 1977]), it is important to discuss this programme in some detail.

PET differs from most group intervention programmes in that it was not created specifically for the lower classes, or for families in which children already display severe emotional disturbance. Though more recently PET classes have been held in low-income sections of large cities, it still attracts primarily the middle classes because, instead of being paid to participate (from government funds) or participating at no cost to them (again, from government funds) most parents taught by authorized PET instructors pay a fee, however nominal. This does not detract from its value; it only defines the majority of the population it serves. While PET techniques are available through a book marketed to the public (Gordon 1970), it is assumed that it is primarily the middle-class public who buy it.

Nevertheless, PET does bring the child into the problem-solving process, as parents are trained in specific communication techniques. As true of the interventions for parents of normal lower-class children, PET is a preventive programme designed to offer 'help to parents before their children develop behavioural problems and before the parent–child relationship deteriorates' (*New Training Models for Delinquency Prevention* 1976, p. 4). Drawing from his training as a Rogerian therapist, Gordon seeks to help families cope with life's problems by teaching them three major strategies. One of these, called 'active listening' engages the parents to reflect their child's feelings at the moment, and to then feed back in a non-judging and accepting way, how they interpret those feelings. Another strategy parents learn is to communicate 'I' messages, such as 'I'm too tired to play with you', instead of 'You' messages, such as 'You are being a pest'. The third, and perhaps most stressed strategy incorporates what Gordon calls the 'No-Lose Problem Solving Method', which includes suggestions to help a child discuss the problem, to enumerate different possible solutions, and to aim at a mutually satisfactory resolution. Implicit in these strategies is that as these are used children will be less likely to engage in unacceptable behaviours, because their self-esteem is not threatened and also because they have participated in the decision-making process.

In their review of PET evaluation research, Rinn and Markle (1977) note a general lack of rigorous, scientific design, leaving the question of programme effectiveness open. Some studies lacked outside observers, leaving possible bias in parents' reports unchecked. Others lacked suitable control groups, making it difficult to attribute any improvement specifically to PET. Examining the studies cited by Rinn and Markle and the 1979 list distributed by Effectiveness Training Incorporated, it seems that, despite methodological difficulties, some form of attitudinal change (e.g. parents' acceptance of children's behaviours and feelings, parents' confidence in their role, and/or mutual parent–child trust and understanding) was reported by more investigators than not — thus reducing the likelihood that such change occurred merely by chance.

Although the focus of the standard PET programme stresses 'modifying the parent rather than the child', the goal being 'to help parents become more effective as "therapeutic agents" for their own children' (*New Training Models for Delinquency Prevention* 1976, p. 5), three studies have examined the effect of this training on the behaviour of children — with two of these having also provided the children with some type of intervention. However, Rinn and Markle note that Miles's (1974) data of teacher-rated behaviours of potential high-school drop-outs did not show improvement beyond that of non-trained groups, even with the addition of positive verbal reinforcement to children who evaluated and considered ways to perpetuate the positive aspects of their present situation. While Andelin (1975) found learning disabled and/or emotionally disturbed children did not improve behaviour in either parent or parent–child PET groups, Dubey, *et al.* (1977) did find PET parent training to have significantly reduced hyperactivity, but no more than in children of parents exposed to classical behaviour modification techniques. Parents in both groups observed reduction in the incidence and severity of other problems named, but this reduction favoured children whose parents were trained in the Behaviour rather than in the PET group.

Importantly, Dubey, *et al.* also report that more parents in the Behaviour than in the PET group judged the workshops to be relevant to their own children's behaviours and that fewer of them dropped out prematurely. This, and the lack of clear behaviour change in these studies which can be specifically attributed to PET, may well have occurred because PET was designed as a preventive rather than as a treatment programme and may therefore be relevant for more typical everyday parent–child conflicts and behavioural difficulties than those exhibited by potential school drop-outs, or by diagnostically disturbed and/or hyperactive children. Although PET parents who tell their children 'I'm too tired to play with you' (I-message) are clearly communicating in a way which is less damaging to their self-esteem than saying 'You are being a pest' (You-message), the difficulties may lie in assuming that the children are already sensitive to, and concerned with, the other person's feelings. Perhaps when children are brought into the mutual problem-solving process (to the satisfaction of both parent and child), it is also assumed that the children have developed the cognitive skills necessary both to appreciate the other's perspective of the problem and to enable the children to help solve it.

Despite inconsistencies in the results of these studies and the research-design problems inherent in some of them, the overall picture for group educational programmes for parents (including PET) is generally encouraging. As Dubey, *et al.* point out, they provide a model which is potentially 'more likely to develop competence in dealing with the problems of child management *and over a longer period of time than the individual treatment model which depends on* the continued ingenuity of a child management specialist' (p. 10, my italics).

Child-focused training

Given the potential value of the group educational model, another approach is to identify those thinking skills which are associated with social adjustment and interpersonal competence. Once these skills are confirmed, parents can be trained to help their children learn these skills and how to use them when problems come up. With the idea of enhancing social skills development early in the child's life, myself and my colleague, George Spivack, began to investigate those thinking skills which would distinguish behaviourally adjusted from more aberrant children aged 4–5 years.

Interpersonal thinking skills of young children

Our research with 4- and 5-year-olds included relatively normal children, who in the preschools and kindergartens they attend varied in the extent to which they displayed behavioural difficulties with peers and adults.

In seven separate studies (reviewed in Spivack, *et al.* 1976), we have consistently found that regardless of IQ, general verbal ability, sex of the child and socioeconomic level, the single best cognitive predictor of teacher-rated school behavioural adjustment in this age group is *alternative solution thinking*. As measured by the Preschool Interpersonal Problem Solving test, or PIPS test (Shure and Spivack 1974), we learned that children who were capable of generating multiple options to peer-type problems (such as wanting a toy another child has) and to adult-type problems (such as how to keep mother from being angry after having damaged property) were also less likely to display behaviours defining impulsiveness. For example, better problem solvers were, relative to poor ones, more able to wait their turn when interacting with peers and less nagging and demanding of adults. They were less overemotional when things did not go their way and usually less physically and/or verbally aggressive. Good problem solvers were also less likely to have exhibited shyness, timidity or fear of peers and/or figures of authority — behaviours which inhibit appropriate display of feelings, ability to stand up for their rights, or expression of even normal amounts of aggression. In addition, good problem solvers were perceived by their teachers as more sociable, especially in the extent to which they appeared to be concerned and/or offered help to their peers in distress, and to how much they were liked and sought out by others. (For a complete rating scale see Shure and Spivack 1974.)

A second skill intimately associated with healthy adjustment is consequential thinking, or ability to anticipate what might happen if a child grabs a toy from another, or takes something from an adult without first asking. As measured by the 'What Happens Next Game', or WHNG (Shure and Spivack 1975a), we learned that while better-adjusted children could think of more potential consequences to interpersonal acts than could the more poorly adjusted, this thinking skill highlights most particularly the deficiencies of the inhibited. Perhaps any awareness of consequences does not stop impulsive youngsters because other than ask (for a toy), which is often refused, these children cannot, or do not, think of what else to do. Instead of pursuing a new course of action they may well create a new problem with their quick and sure way to get it 'now'. Consistent with this, our recent pilot study has suggested that impulsive children are also particularly unaware, or at best unconcerned with, other people's feelings; they also appear to be unaware that others may feel differently than they do about something. However cognizant of the consequences, any recognition or concern that their actions may lead to their own happiness at another's expense is apparently disregarded.

Sensitivity to, and appeciation of, others' feelings — skills called role taking or perspective taking — were found to be somewhat more important to inhibited than to impulsive youngsters. However, inhibited children do not seem able to conceptualize solutions or consequences. Perhaps these youngsters have experienced failure so often that they withdraw from people, and from problems that they cannot solve. For some inhibited children any knowledge or sensitivity to feelings without the capability to deal with them may be frightening enough to cause social withdrawal.

Although this is not directly related to behaviour, good problem solvers when shown a picture of people and asked 'What's wrong?' were more likely to state an interpersonal problem (e.g. 'The boy is in the way and his parents can't see the TV'); poor problem solvers would be more likely to state a personal problem (e.g. 'The boy's pants are ripped') or an impersonal one (e.g. 'The TV is broken'). In addition to this cognitive sensitivity to interpersonal problems, good problem solvers were also more able than poor ones to think of what might have led to a problem, thus showing greater appreciation of interpersonal cause-and-effect.

Thus in our population of inner-city 4- and 5-year-olds, those who are deficient in solution thinking apparently may or may not consider the effects of their actions on the feelings or behaviour of others, probably do not recognize the event(s) that led up to the problem and are probably not even aware or concerned about the problem that exists. For impulsive children absorbed in their own needs, what might happen next becomes only secondary, and they continue to pursue their original desire by the limited repertoire of options that they have. Our complete series of studies suggests that cognitive interpersonal sensitivity, causal thinking and perspective-taking may enrich solution and consequential thinking but that of all interpersonal thinking skills measured to date, knowing what else to do (alternative-solution thinking) is the cognitive skill that best prevents, or at least diminishes, continued frustration and subsequent need for impulsive behaviours or withdrawal.

Since educators and clinicians have long believed that if emotional tension could be relieved it would be easier to think straight, it seemed reasonable to believe that if one could think straight it would be easier to relieve emotional tension.

Our next step was to empirically test Spivack's (1973) assumption that the availability of what we came to call Interpersonal Cognitive Problem Solving, or ICPS, skills is an antecedent condition for healthy social adjustment. Systematic training of children by their teachers showed that relative to untrained controls, preschool and kindergarten children could significantly increase their ICPS ability (Shure and Spivack 1979). In support of Spivack's findings, those who most improved in the trained solution and consequential thinking skills were the same children who also most improved in behaviours defining impulsiveness and inhibition, in prosocial concern, and in how well they were liked by their peers (Shure and Spivack 1974, 1975*a*, 1980).

Childrearing, ICPS and social development

If teachers could have a large effect on the ICPS skills and behaviour of young children, we reasoned that effects of training could be still greater if parents were exposed to the intervention as well. Before implementing such a programme we set out to discover how, during everyday life, mothers of inner-city 4-year-olds can and do contribute to their child's ICPS and social development.

Background research

In two studies (Shure and Spivack 1978) we related ICPS and communication skills of poor, black inner-city mothers to the ICPS skills and school-observed behaviour of their children. Using a modified version of the means—ends problem solving (MEPS) test (Platt and Spivack 1975), mothers were asked to tell a story about how they would solve hypothetical mother—child type problems (e.g. Mrs Hill's children are squabbling and she can't think about her dinner) and child—child type problems (e.g. a mother learned that her child has been hitting other children lately, and she feels concerned about this). We discovered that mothers adept at 'means—ends' thinking, that is, who could plan sequenced steps to reach a stated goal, who could anticipate and think of ways to overcome potential obstacles, and who could recognize that goal attainment may take time were, when required to handle genuine problems, more likely to offer suggestions, explain the consequences (induction), and talk to their child about feelings (e.g. 'I feel angry when you do that'). These child-rearing techniques were among the most sophisticated used, and are the same techniques advocated by the researchers and educators who designed the intervention programmes described earlier. Our studies showed that parents who used these techniques did have better problem solvers and better-adjusted children, but only if the child was a girl.

Why not in boys? We're not sure, but as Hoffman (1971) has noted, boys are naturally more resistant to influence than girls, and may be even more so when they do not have fathers (the case in nearly 70 per cent of our youngsters). If, as Hoffman has also noted, mothers are more affectionate to their fatherless girls than to boys and if children adopt parental characteristics more from parents who provide a relatively consistent source of nurturance and reward (e.g. Mussen and Rutherford 1963), young fatherless boys may resist modelling their mother's problem-solving style just as they might resist other forms of influence and discipline.

So where do boys who are no less deficient than girls acquire their problem-solving skills? Fathers do not exert a large effect on the acquisition of such skills in boys. Flaherty (1978), who has confirmed our mother–daughter but not son relationships has also learned that even in parentally intact homes fathers' style of handling problems with their children has little influence on the problem-solving skills of either their daughters or their sons. Could, as Radin (1973) suggests, the amount of paternal restrictiveness in the lower classes overshadow nurturance? If too little nurturance is given by lower-class fathers to their sons, perhaps they resist their fathers' demands, thus leaving them with no greater problem-solving modelling agents than boys who have no father at all.

To complicate matters further it is not even clear where boys in the middle classes learn their problem-solving skills. Howie (unpublished observations) found significant relationships between both mothers' *and* fathers' childrearing attitudes and preschool daughters' (but not sons') alternative-solution thinking. Encouragement to verbalize feelings or to express oneself freely was associated with better problem-solving thinking. Further, better problem-solving girls had fathers who were less control-oriented in their discipline. In boys, none of the correlations between fathers' childrearing attitudes and sons' problem-solving thinking were significant. The only significant maternal correlation indicated that better problem solving among sons was related to mother's proneness to control behaviour harshly, a finding similar to our own in lower-class fatherless boys (Shure and Spivack 1975a).

Whatever the case, clear communication in the form of instructions, suggestions and induction does not seem to affect the interpersonal thinking skills and behaviour in boys in the same way it appears to in girls (see Shure and Spivack 1978). Whatever the eventual truths regarding the current 'natural' childrearing precursors of interpersonal problem-solving thinking, we set out to discover if ICPS skills and behaviour of both boys *and* girls could be enhanced if the mother were trained in problem-solving techniques of childrearing.

The ICPS approach to childrearing

Although *what* a person thinks is not claimed to be irrelevant to adjustment, we believe that a wide repertoire of options can help to choose an effective solution if the first one(s) should fail. We believe that the *process* of thinking is more critical to adjustment than the content of specific solutions conceived, and it is this premise that underlies the ICPS approach to childrearing.

Our training strategies grew out of what we learned from what children actually do and say, from our above-described teacher-training research, and from our test results. It became clear that adjusted children, just as aberrant ones, could think of forceful ways to obtain a toy (e.g. 'Grab it', 'Hit him') and would, on occasion, carry them out. The difference was that adjusted children could also think of more non-forceful ways (e.g. 'I'll be your friend', 'Say please', 'You can play with my truck'). While children did not always do what they said could be done (when specifically asked), our findings suggest that there is a general process, or style of evaluating multiple options, that relates to a pattern of well-adjusted behaviour. Given this, we would not try to inhibit any particular content of thought. Rather, we would help ICPS-deficient children think about what they do and consider other ways to solve the problem.

For children, our strategies were designed to help them develop the habit of generating *different* ways, not adult-valued good ways to satisfy their needs and cope with frustration. Encouraging children to think of their own solutions to problems and consequences to acts would, in our view, add to their understanding of what they do in interpersonal situations. If, for example, a child hits another or grabs a toy, he is asked why he did that, what the other child did or said, and whether or not his action was a good idea. On the basis of his response the child may be reminded that hitting is *one* thing he can do and then be asked if he can think of something different he can do to solve the problem.

Helping children to think like this can also make a difference when problems come up with their parents. One child wanted her mother to read her a story. When her mother told her she was busy and would read to her later, the child whined 'But I want it now!' Unable to wait, the child became more demanding and her mother became angry. Whether or not this girl foresaw the consequences of her action, her lack of solution thinking led her to repeat her demands, which created a new problem (mother's anger) and thus intensified her frustration.

If children who are poor problem solvers often experience frustration and failure their parents may also experience frustration and failure when problems come up with their children. In our pretraining interviews, we learned that many were just as preoccupied with their needs as their children were with their own. When asked how they generally handled typical problems that came up during the day, several offered dialogues similar to these:

<table>
<tr><td align="center">(I)</td><td align="center">(II)</td></tr>
<tr><td>

Child: Peter hit me today.
Mother: Hit him back.
   C: He'd punch me in the nose.
   M: Every time he hits you, hit him back. I don't want you to be so timid.
   C: But I'm afraid.
   M: If you don't learn to defend yourself, kids will keep on hitting you.
   C: OK.

</td><td>

C: Danny knocked me down.
M: What did you do then?
C: I hit him back.
M: You shouldn't hit back. Hitting is not nice. You might hurt someone. It's better to tell the teacher.
C: Then he'll call me a tattletale.
M: If you don't tell the teacher, he'll keep on hitting you.
C: OK.

</td></tr>
</table>

(From Shure and Spivack 1978, p. 118.)

These mothers gave different advice to their children. But they used the same approach.

Though both children thought about a consequence of their mother's suggested solution, these mothers ignored the child's view and suggested consequences of their own. Instead of encouraging their children to think through the problem, these mothers did the thinking for them. In the end, these children no longer had to decide what to do, only worry about how to do it (or keep their mother from learning that they hadn't). Preoccupied with their own point of view, these mothers ignored their children's perception of the problem or why they were hit in the first place. As many mothers told us, their children came back a few days later with the same problem (no matter what their advice had been).

To help mothers guide their child to develop a problem-solving process of thinking, strategies for parents were designed to:

(1) increase sensitivity that their child's view may differ from their own;
(2) lead to a realization that thinking about what is happening may, in the long run, be more beneficial than immediate action to stop it;

(3) increase awareness that there is more than one way to solve a problem; and

(4) provide a model of problem-solving thinking — a thinking parent might inspire a child to think.

As mothers were trained in problem-solving thinking skills they, in turn, taught their children lessons from a sequenced day-by-day programme script (in Shure and Spivack 1978), as demonstrated and role played in ten weekly workshops (Shure 1979).

Because many parents and their children were relatively deficient in their ICPS skills at the start, skills we judged to be prerequisite to the final skills to be learned were included. As the mother helped her child think about his own and others' feelings and how to consider the effects of his actions upon others, she was also guided to think about her feelings and how what *she* does affects others (including her child). As a mother guided her child to find out what led up to a problem (e.g. 'Why he was hit') the mother also thought about how to find out what happened. In learning that her own view of a problem (e.g. 'You must learn to share your toys') may be different from her child's ('But I did share; now I want my truck back!') she also helps her child recognize viewpoints. And, as a mother guides her child to think of solutions to problems relevant to him, she also thinks of solutions to problems relevant to her (particularly when a child creates a problem affecting her, such as 'Mike won't do what I ask him to, lately'). Just as the child was never told solutions to problems or consequences of acts, neither were the mothers. The value was not on *what* they thought, but that they did so.

ICPS training effects

Relative to untrained controls matched for age, sex, behavioural adjustment and ICPS ability, mother-trained, black lower-class boys *and* girls significantly improved in ICPS ability, especially solution skills, and in teacher-rated behaviours defining impulsiveness and inhibition. Mothers, relative to their controls (equated for initial ICPS and communication skills) improved in their own ability to solve hypothetical problems as well as in their use of a problem-solving style of communication when problems arose.

Mothers' improved ability to solve hypothetical adult problems (such as how to keep a friend from being angry after showing up too late to go to the cinema) did *not* relate to her child's improved ICPS skills, but her ability to solve hypothetical problems about children (or about children and their parents) did. Also, we discovered that mothers who best learned to plan step-by-step means to solve a child-related problem (such as how a mother could get her child to stop being a bully), who could see potential obstacles (that problem solving is not always smooth sailing), and who were likely to allow a hypothetical child to generate solutions and consequences were the same mothers who were most likely to apply problem-solving techniques of communication for real problems. These relationships suggest that increasing mother's ability to think about these kinds of problems is intimately related to how she guides her child to solve real problems as they arise, and together both have an important effect on the child's ICPS skills.

After training a child who had been hit had a different conversation with his mother:

> *Child:* Mommy, Tommy hit me.
> *Mother:* Why did he hit you? *(Mother elicits child's view of the problem.)*
> *C:* I don't know.
> *M:* He might have hit you because . . .
> *C:* He was mad.
> *M:* Why was he mad? *(Mother guides child to think of other's point of view.)*
> *C:* 'Cause I took his truck.
> *M:* Is that why he hit you?
> *C:* Yep!
> *M:* Grabbing is one way to get that truck. Can you think of something different to do so he won't hit you? *(Mother guides child to think of solutions.)*
> *C:* I could tell him I'd just play a little while.
> *M:* That's a different idea.

(From Shure and Spivack 1975*b*, p. 7.)

With this kind of communication (which we call problem-solving 'dialoguing') the mother gained information that her first dialogue would not have allowed. With the child having gained the habit of thinking of alternatives, this mother could elicit more solutions as back-up should the first one be unsuccessful. Importantly, not only did children learn to think of how to get what they wanted when they could have it, they also learned to cope with the frustration when they could not. In one example, a child wanted to go to a friend's house after dinner:

Child: Mom, can I go to play with Tracy?
Mother: Not now, It's too late.
    C: I'll come straight back. We just want to play for a little while.
    M: Why do you think I don't want you to go now? *(Mother guides child to consider her viewpoint.)*
    C: It's almost bedtime.
    M: Yes, that's one reason. What's another reason?
    C: It's very dark.
    M: Yes, that too. So how do you think I'll feel if you go and play with Tracy now? *(Mother does not tell how she feels, but encourages child to think it through.)*
    C: Mad.
    M: Can you think of something different to do now?
    C: I'll play with my toys.
    M: You thought of that all by yourself.

If nagging and demanding is often a child's *solution* to a problem, and not the problem itself, emotional confrontation can be avoided by both the parent and child recognizing the problem and each other's point of view. Had this mother suggested, 'Why don't you play with your toys?' the child would probably have answered, 'But I don't want to play with my toys!' increasing, no doubt, both the mother's and the child's frustration. Instead, this child felt good about her 'own' idea, and any potential power play became unnecessary.

The words, however, are not enough; the whole approach matters. To guide a child to think about a problem takes time, patience and warmth. However, this is not to say a parent should never get angry with their children. Anger is a problem with which children must learn to cope, *if* they are encouraged to think that way — and if anger and emotional outbursts are not predominant.

While mothers' improved ICPS and communication skills affected change in their children's solution and consequential skills, co-variance analyses suggested it was change in the children's ICPS skills which had the largest direct effect on their behaviour. As in our teacher-training research, alternative-solution thinking again emerged as most strongly related to behaviour before training and most receptive to change after it, and it was change in this skill that most directly related to change in behaviour.

It was particularly gratifying that girls *and* boys could benefit equally from ICPS training by their mothers (given that at pretest, statistical relationships were significant for girls only). We believe that this may have happened because trained mothers acquired thinking skills above and beyond those which even the best problem solvers exhibited initially. As previously noted, before training better problem-solving mothers offered solutions and sometimes explained consequences, whereas relatively ICPS-deficient mothers more often used abrupt commands without explanation. If, as also noted earlier, boys are naturally more resistant to modelling ICPS skills of their mothers, they may be less resistant to it when guided, then freed to think for themselves.

The results might have been due to the extra attention mothers gave to their children. In this regard, children whose mothers received ICPS training improved more than an earlier trained group whose mothers administered the programme script to their children (requiring the same amount of attention) and also learned to 'dialogue' but whose training did not include problem-solving thinking of their own (see Shure and Spivack 1978). If the child's improvement were due to mere attention the change in the first group would have equalled that of the second. Perhaps the second group of mothers not only gained more insight about the concepts they taught to their children but also a greater sensitivity to the sensations their children experienced as they learned these concepts. While both of these mother-trained groups improved more than non-trained controls the findings suggest that greater ICPS and behavioural effects on children occur when mothers and their children learn relevant interpersonal thinking skills.

Importantly, children trained at home improved their behaviour as observed in school, validating not only the behaviour change (the teachers were unaware of the training procedures and its goals) but also the approach; the behaviour change occurred in an environment different from that in which the training took place. If our theory of adjustment is correct, perhaps this happened because children learned *how* to think, and could generalize their newly acquired skills to more than one situation. That ICPS and behaviour change in children trained by their mothers was similar to that of children trained by their teachers is particularly encouraging. It is important to know that inner-city lower-class mothers, many of whom were ICPS-deficient at the start, could improve not only *their* abilities but those of their child in only 3 months.

The validity of ICPS training for the middle classes has recently been confirmed by Wowkanech (personal communication). Two groups of 4-year-olds were trained, one group receiving the ICPS approach, the other a programme in which teachers suggested solutions, modelled how to carry them out and explained the consequences. Observed by independent raters (research staff who were unaware of group composition), her results clearly showed that during conflict, ICPS-trained children spontaneously generated their own solutions to the problem and turned to a different one if the conflict was not resolved. On the other hand, tactics of the modelling groups, once training had ceased, more often reverted to those previously used — such as hitting, grabbing or commands. In handling conflict, the important issue is that these children tried more than one way to deal with it less often.

ICPS after age five

Interviews with the parents of 6–16-year-olds in both the middle and lower social classes have provided insight about how unusual the problem-solving approach is. Although the content of particular problems and what parents do or say may differ, the extent to which parents encourage children to think does not change because the children get older or because they belong to the middle classes.

One middle-class 15-year-old boy was angry with his brother (age 12) for taking his bike without permission. He told his father what happened.

Father: Well, don't get all excited about it. He'll be back in a little while.

 Child: But dad, I want my bike *now*! Why can't he ride his own bike?

    F: I'll tell him not take your bike again without your permission.

    C: But dad, he never asks, and he always takes it. He takes the bike and doesn't come back for 2 hours, and you never do anything about it! Next time . . .

    F: (Interrupts) Don't you talk to *me* like that!

    C: I'm just going to take something of his and hide it.

    F: You'll be sorry if you do that! If you would allow him to borrow your bike sometimes, he wouldn't take it like that.

C: I don't care. I don't want him using my bike.
F: I heard you. Now drop it. I told you I'll talk to him about it.

This father (however unaware of it), tries to relieve his son of any further thought about the problem ('I'll tell him not to'). When the son offers a solution of his own the father, instead of encouraging him to evaluate that solution, simply gets angry, offers his own idea, and then returns to his original plan to solve the problem for him.

The effect of problem-solving communication (or lack of it) on the problem-solving skills and behaviour of older children is relatively unexplored. In one study, Herman (1978) observed mothers teaching their child a magic trick and then noticed how both presented it to the experimenter. He found retarded 9–11-year-olds whose mothers were generally supportive and allowed them to make their own decisions to be better interpersonal-problem solvers than those whose mothers directed their children's actions, or interfered with their course of action. Examining the effect of parents on perspective-taking skills of 6- and 7-year-olds, Bearison and Cassel (1975) have learned that mothers who appealed to human needs, thoughts and feelings had children who were more sensitive to the perspective of the listener while communicating than were children whose mothers appealed to rules or merely demanded conformity.

If, as we believe, appreciation of the viewpoint of others enhances problem-solving skills by enriching the nature and range of solutions from which to choose, it also seems reasonable to assume that the content of those solutions would be interactional. Although I know of no such studies with older children, the findings of Jones, *et al.* (1980) on 4-year-olds may have important implications in other age groups. Regardless of social class, restrictive mothers (concerned with rules and conformity) had children who offered evasion strategies to the PIPS-mother-type problem (how to keep mother from being angry after having damaged property); strategies that Jones, *et al.* interpret as requiring no attempt to deal with the thoughts, feelings and needs of the other (e.g. 'hide', 'hide the broken flower pot', 'say I didn't do it'). In the light of Bearison and Cassel's findings, it is interesting that Jones, *et al.* found that more-nurturant mothers (who were warm, involved with the children, and recognized their desires and emotional needs) had children who offered more solutions of personal appeal and negotiation (e.g. 'Mom, don't be mad', or in the peer-type story, 'I'll give the truck back'); solutions that include reciprocal recognition of others' thoughts, feelings and wishes.

How the interrelationships of childrearing style, parent and child perspective taking, and both the process (quantity) and structure (quality) of problem-solving skills affect each other and the child's social adjustment at various ages could provide an extremely fruitful framework for research.

With implications for childrearing in mind, our own work and that of others have identified specific ICPS skills associated with social adjustment at various ages, skills which have clear implications for extending parent ICPS training to a wide variety of age groups.

As reviewed by Spivack, *et al.* (1976), alternative-solution thinking and perspective taking (see Shantz 1975) continue to be important skills for adjustment throughout adolescence.

Elias (1978) discovered that means–ends thinking in children by the age of 6, when asking only for step-by-step means to reach a stated goal, has provided 'meaningful predictors of independent social problem solving behaviour as perceived by peers on sociometrics' (p. 185). The ability to anticipate obstacles and the recognition that problem solving may take time (completing the elements of total means–ends thinking) do not appear to relate to adjustment until the age of 9 or 10, and are particularly relevant to social competence during adolescence. When asked for a story about how a child can make friends in a new neighbourhood, a well-adjusted 11-year-old boy gave this one:

> 'First Al got talking to the leader. He found out the kids liked basketball but Al didn't know how to play. When Al got to know the leader better he asked him to get the kids down to the skating rink. The kids went and saw him practicing shooting goals. So the kids asked him, "Would you teach us how to do that?" So he did and they organized two teams and the kids liked that and Al had lots of friends.'   (Spivack, *et al.* 1976, p. 66.)

This child invented a story wherein the first mean, talking to the leader, uncovered an obstacle — the kids liked a game that Al didn't know how to play. The obstacle was overcome by stimulating interest in another game (ice-hockey) that Al did know how to play. A recognition of time was manifested by the statement 'When Al got to know the leader better'.

Regardless of social class, relatively impatient children tend to invent stories suggesting that thinking moves immediately to goal attainment with insufficient consideration of how to get there and insufficient awareness of obstacles that might have to be overcome. Typical stories describe the child meeting others in the playground and then being introduced by a chain of other children, culminating in the group. The remainder of these stories describe how they play together 'after they are friends'. My most recent study (Shure 1980) has shown that 10-year-olds who were judged both by teacher ratings and peer sociometrics to be well liked (by their peers) showed the most sophisticated means–ends skills with regard to this story about making friends. However relevant the content identification may be (being liked is apparently no accident), stories of getting even with a peer for having made a nasty remark also relate to prosocial behaviours, especially the extent to which a child is sensitive to, and concerned about, a peer who is experiencing distress. That *content* of the story should include social and not-so-social goals further supports the belief that the *process* of thought is important.

Our recent study with 10-year-olds has also shown that when specifically asked what might happen, ability to invent multiple consequences relates to behaviour: not only to impulsiveness and inhibition but also, as in younger children, to being liked and concerned for others. This ability also related to a new measure, that of how much they were perceived by teachers and peers to be 'good leaders'. A more sophisticated process of consequential thinking, that of spontaneously weighing pros and cons, does not appear to be important in this age group (Larcen, *et al.* 1972), but does by adolescence (Spivack and Levine 1963). For example, a child is told that someone is trying to decide whether to go to a party or study for an examination and is then asked to tell what is going on in that person's mind. The spontaneous tendency to simultaneously weigh pros *and* cons, e.g. 'If I go to the party, I'll have more fun, but my mother will be mad and I might fail my exam', may be developmentally too sophisticated before adolescence.

Interpersonal cause and effect and cognitive sensitivity to interpersonal problems do not appear to relate to adjustment in any age group from preschool to adolescence (at least as measured to date). Because these skills may well include concepts prerequisite to problem-solving ability (as discussed earlier), it appears to be fruitful to retain them as part of the total ICPS-training package.

To date, ICPS training of parents and their older children has not been conducted. However, such training by teachers of 8–10-year-olds has been effective (e.g. Elardo and Caldwell 1979), though behaviour change may take a little longer (Gesten, *et al.* unpublished observations). Although it is undoubtedly advantageous to start at the earliest age possible, it seems reasonable to assume that ICPS training for parents and children would also benefit older children. For these youngsters the additional guidance of means–ends skills would be compatible with their developmental level of skill acquisition, both as part of the formal lessons and in 'dialogues' (e.g. 'What's the next step?' [sequenced means]; 'Is there anything that could stop you?' [obstacle]; 'How long do you think that will take?' [time recognition]).

Final thoughts

If interpersonal cognitive problem-solving skills can add to our understanding of the quality of social adjustment, it also appears that applying them does not generalize from being told, or shown the way. In this vein, one mother said 'It [the programme] doesn't tell me *what* to do. It helps me think better when I have my own problems.' Another added 'James puts the pictures on his wall. He asks *me* questions about them. One day I heard him telling Whipple (a puppet) *all* the things he could do so Allie (another puppet) would play with him. I couldn't believe my ears.' Mothers also received the programme enthusiastically because it does not require a change of childrearing goals (just in how to accomplish them), or a shift in values of parents in either lower- or middle-class social groups. Though a day-by-day programme script is provided for those who need or desire it, parents are free to create games suitable for their own children (within programme goals), allowing flexibility. One mother, who valued the latter, put it best: 'After a while I could make up my own games. That made me feel smart.'

A question remains as to how soon children could benefit from the ICPS approach to childrearing. Could training parents to use a process of problem-solving thinking affect their communication skills with children under the age of 4? Though their goal was not specifically to help children later solve interpersonal problems, Lambie (1976) did guide parents to think of their own ideas about what to do when, for example, their baby was uncomfortable and crying when strapped into a car seat. This approach holds real promise because right from the start these parents may have an effect on later interpersonal problem-solving skills and social adjustment of their children.

While we make no claim that the ICPS approach is the only way to optimize social development and interpersonal competence, it clearly adds another option for techniques from which to choose. If social skills embrace thought as well as deed the ICPS approach helps us appreciate how the way people think can affect what they do.

References

Allen, G., Chinsky, J., Larcen, S., Lochman, J. and Selinger, H. (1976). *Community Psychology and the Schools: A Behaviorally Oriented Multilevel Preventive Approach*. Hillsdale, N.J.: Earlbaum.

Andelin, S. (1975). *The Effects of Concurrently Teaching Parents and their Children with Learning Adjustment Problems the Principles of Parent Effectiveness Training*. Ph.D. thesis, Utah State University.

Baldwin, A. and Baldwin, C. (1976). *The Study of Interpersonal Interaction in Disturbed Children. Interim Report*. The Grant Foundation.

Baumrind, D. (1967). Child care practices anteceding three patterns of pre-school behavior. *Gen. Psychol. Monographs* 75, 44−88.

Bearison, D. J. and Cassell, T. Z. (1975). Cognitive decentration and social codes: Communicative effectiveness in young children from differing family contexts. *Dev. Psychol.* 11, 29−36.

Becker, W. C. (1964). Consequences of different kinds of parental discipline. *In* Hoffman, M. L. and Hoffman, L. W. (eds). *Review of Child Development Research*. New York: Russell Sage Foundation, vol. 1.

Bronfennbrenner, U. (1974). *Is Early Intervention Effective? A Report on Longitudinal Evaluations of Preschool Programs*. Washington, D.C.: Office of Child Development, Departments of Health, Education and Welfare, vol. 2.

Cole, R. (1981). Family interaction and peer acceptance. In preparation.

Combs, M. L. and Slaby, D. A. (1979). Social skills training with children. *In* Lahey, B. and Kazdin, A. (eds). *Advances in Clinical Child Psychology*. New York: Plenum, vol. 1.

Dubey, D. R., Kaufman, K. F. and O'Leary, S. G. (1977). *Behavioral and Reflective Parent Training for Hyperactive Children: A Comparison*. Presented at the meetings of the American Psychological Association, San Francisco, August.

Elardo, P. T. and Caldwell, B. M. (1979). The effects of an experimental social development program on children in the middle childhood period. *Psychol. Schools* 16, 93−100.

Elias, M. J. (1978). *The Development of a Theory-Based Measure of How Children Understand and Attempt to Resolve Problematic Social Situations*. M.Sc. thesis, University of Connecticut.

Flaherty, E. (1978). *Parental Influence on Children's Social Cognition*.

Washington, D.C.: National Institute of Mental Health, Final Summary Report No. 29033.

Gesten, E. L., Rains, M. H., Rapkin, B. D., Weissberg, R. P., Flores de Apodaca, R., Cowen, E. L. and Bowen, R. (1981). Training children in social problem solving competencies: a first and second look. *Am. J. Comm. Psychol.* In preparation.

Gordon, T. (1970). *Parent Effectiveness Training (PET).* New York: Peter H. Wyden, Inc.

Gordon, T. (1977). Parent Effectiveness Training: A Preventive Program and its Delivery System. *In* Albee, G. W. and Joffe, J. M. (eds). *The Primary Prevention of Psychopathology. Vol. I: The Issues.* Hanover, N. H.: University Press of New England.

Heinicke, C. M. (1976). Aiding 'at risk' children through psychoanalytic social work with parents. *Am. J. Orthopsychiatr.* 46, 89–103.

_____ (1977). *Changes in the Preschool Child as a Function of Change in the Parent–Child Relationship.* Presented at the meeting of the Society for Research in Child Development, New Orleans, March.

Herman, M. S. (1978). *The Mother–Child Interaction, Social Competence and Locus of Control as Correlates of the Interpersonal Competence of Educable Mentally Retarded and Normal Children.* M.Sc. thesis, Wayne State University.

Hoffman, M. L. (1963). Parent discipline and the child's consideration for others. *Child Dev.* 34, 573–88.

_____ (1970*a*). Conscience, personality, and socialization techniques. *Hum. Dev.* 13, 90–126.

_____ (1970*b*). Moral development. *In* Mussen, P. H. (ed.). *Carmichael's Manual of Child Psychology.* New York: Wiley, vol. II.

_____ (1971). Father-absence and conscience development. *Dev. Psychol.* 4, 400–6.

Hoffman, M. L. and Saltzstein, H. D. (1967). Parent discipline and the child's moral development. *J. Personality Soc. Psychol.* 5, 45–57.

Howie, R. D. (1981). The relationship between interpersonal problem solving ability of 4-year-olds and parental values and attitudes. In preparation.

Johnson, D. L., Kahn, A. J. and Leler, H. (1976). *Houston Parent–Child Development Center. Final Report.* DHEW-90-C-379. Houston: Office of Child Development. (DHEW No. 90-C-379.)

Jones, D. C., Rickel, A. U. and Smith, R. L. (1980). Maternal child-rearing practices and social problem solving strategies among preschoolers. *J. Dev. Psychol.* 16, 241–2.

Lambie, D. Z. (1975–6). *Parents and Educators: Experts and Equals.* Ypsilanti: High/Scope Educational Research Foundation, pp. 22–6. (The High/Scope Report.)

Larcen, S. W., Spivack, G. and Shure, M. (1972). *Problem-Solving Thinking and Adjustment among Dependent–Neglected Preadolescents.* Presented at the meeting of the Eastern Psychological Association, Boston, April.

Mahoney, M. (1974). *Cognition and Behavior Modification.* Cambridge, Mass.: Ballinger.

Meichenbaum, D. (1977). *Cognitive-Behavior Modification: An Integrative Approach.* New York: Plenum Press.

Miles, J. M. H. (1974). *A Comparative Analysis of the Effectiveness of Verbal Reinforcement Group Counseling and Parent Effectiveness Training on Certain Behavioral Aspects of Potential Dropouts*. Ph.D. thesis, Auburn University.

Mussen, P. and Rutherford, E. (1963). Parent–child relations and parental personality in relation to young children's sex-role preferences. *Child Dev.* 34, 589–607.

New training models for delinquency prevention: Position paper (1976). Effectiveness Training Incorporated, Solana Beach, Cal.

Parker, R. J. (ed.) (1972). *The Preschool in Action: Exploring Early Childhood Programs*. Boston: Allyn and Bacon.

Platt, J. J. and Spivack, G. (1975). *Manual for the Means–Ends–Problem-Solving Procedure*. Philadelphia: Department of Mental Health Sciences, Hahnemann Medical College and Hospital.

Radin, N. (1972). Three degrees of maternal involvement in a preschool program: Impact on mothers and children. *Child Dev.* 43, 1355–64.

_____ (1973). Observed paternal behaviors as antecedents of intellectual functioning in young boys. *Dev. Psychol.* 8, 369–76.

Rinn, R. C. and Markle, A. (1977). Parent Effectiveness Training: A review. *Psychol. Rep.* 41, 95–109.

Schaefer, E. S. (1977). Professional paradigms in programs for parents and children. *In* Schroeder, C. S. (Chairman). *Parenting: Training, Problems and Intervention Methods*. Symposium presented at the American Psychological Association, San Francisco, August.

Sears, R. R., Macoby, E. E. and Levin, H. (1957). *Patterns of Child Rearing*. New York: Harper and Row.

Shantz, C. U. (1975). The development of social cognition. *In* Hetherington, E. M. (ed.). *Review of Child Development Research*. Chicago: University of Chicago Press, vol. 5.

Shure, M. B. (1979). Training children to solve interpersonal problems: A preventive mental health program. *In* Muñoz, Snowden, L. R. and Kelly, J. G. (eds). *Social and Psychological Research in Community Settings*. San Francisco: Jossey-Bass.

_____ (1980). *Interpersonal Problem Solving in Ten-Year-Olds*. Washington, D.C.: National Institute of Mental Health. No. MH-27741.

Shure, M. B. and Spivack, G. (1974). *Preschool Interpersonal Problem Solving (PIPS) Test: Manual*. Philadelphia: Department of Mental Health Sciences, Hahnemann Medical College and Hospital.

_____ and _____ (1975a). *A Mental Health Program for Pre-School and Kindergarten Children, and A Mental Health Program for Mothers of Young Children: An Interpersonal Problem-Solving Approach Toward Social Adjustment. A Comprehensive Report of Research and Training*. Washington, D.C.: National Institute of Mental Health, No. MH-20372.

_____ and _____ (1975b). *Training Mothers to Help their Children Solve Real-Life Problems*. Presented at the meeting of the Society for Research in Child Development, Denver, March.

_____ and _____ (1978). *Problem Solving Techniques in Childrearing*. San Francisco: Jossey-Bass.

_____ and _____ (1979). Interpersonal cognitive problem solving and primary prevention: programming for preschool and kindergarten children. *J. Clin. Child Psychol.* 8, 89–94.

_____ and _____ (1980). Interpersonal problem solving as a mediator of behavioral adjustment in preschool and kindergarten children. *J. Appl. Dev. Psychol.* 1, 29–44.

Slaby, D. A. (1981). *Day Treatment and Parent Training Programs.* In preparation.

Spivack, G. (1973). *A Conception of Healthy Human Functioning. Research and Evaluation Report.* Philadelphia: Department of Mental Health Sciences, Hahnemann Medical College and Hospital.

Spivack, G. and Levine, M. (1963). *Self-Regulation in Acting-Out and Normal Adolescents.* Washington, D.C.: National Institute of Health. Report M-4531.

Spivack, G., Platt, J. J. and Shure, M. B. (1976). *The Problem Solving Approach to Adjustment.* San Francisco: Jossey-Bass.

Spivack, G. and Shure, M. B. (1974). *Social Adjustment of Young Children: A Cognitive Approach to Solving Real-Life Problems.* San Francisco: Jossey-Bass.

Wittes, G. and Radin, N. (1969a). *Helping Your Child To Learn: The Learning Through Play Approach.* San Rafael, Cal.: Dimensions Publishing Company.

_____ and _____ (1969b). *Helping Your Child To Learn: The Nurturance Approach.* San Rafael, Cal.: Dimensions Publishing Company.

_____ and _____ (1969c). *Helping Your Child To Learn: The Reinforcement Approach.* San Rafael, Cal.: Dimensions Publishing Company.

_____ and _____ (1971). Two approaches to group work with parents in a compensatory preschool program. *Soc. Work* 16, 42–50.

7 Social competence and mental health

MICHAEL ARGYLE

Introduction

Everybody knows that many mental patients are socially inadequate and difficult to deal with. However, theories of mental disorder have usually regarded these attributes as a minor consequence of other kinds of disturbance — e.g. sexual, cognitive, physiological. Perhaps interpersonal difficulties play a more important role for some kinds of mental patients, in which case social skills training might be a valuable form of treatment for them.

There are now fairly detailed research findings about the social behaviour of mental patients, and we can see which aspects of social performance have failed. Such failures of social competence may be the main cause of mental disturbance. The chain of events could be like this example: a young man has no sisters and attends a boys' school — he does not acquire the skills of dealing with girls and becomes homosexual; this leads to social rejection, which in turn gives rise to depression and anxiety. Alternatively, the failure of social performance could be due to other features of the personality, such as cognitive failure or acute anxiety; again, social incompetence results in rejection and social isolation, and those stresses lead to further deterioration. And there could be complex dynamic processes of the kind described by psychoanalysts, which could lead for example to behaviour which kept other people at a distance.

When failure of social performance is the primary cause a radically different account of mental disorder is being offered: it is not a 'disease', nor need reference be made to 'intrapsychic' disturbances. When failure of social performance is due to other factors, at least part of the psychopathology lies at this new level of social interaction.

Textbooks of psychopathology have kept very quiet about this sphere of behaviour, even though it is usually failure in this sphere which results in the need for treatment (Phillips 1979).

The meaning and assessment of social competence

By social competence I mean the ability, the possession of the necessary skills, to produce the desired effects on other people in social situations. These desired effects may be to persuade the others to buy, learn, recover from neurosis, like or admire the actor and so on. These results are not necessarily in the public interest − skills may be used for social or antisocial purposes. And there is no evidence that social competence is a general factor: a person may be better at one task than another, e.g. interviewing as opposed to lecturing, or in one situation than another, e.g. parties as opposed to committees. In this chapter I shall discuss various forms of social competence. Social skills training (SST) for students and other more or less normal populations has been directed at the skills of dating, making friends and being assertive. SST for mental patients has been aimed at correcting failures of social competence, and also at relieving subjective distress, such as social anxiety.

To find out who needs training, and in what areas, a detailed descriptive assessment is more useful. We want to know, for example, which situations a trainee finds difficult − formal situations, conflicts, meeting strangers, etc., and which situations he is inadequate in, even though he does not report them as difficult. And we want to find out what he is doing wrong: failure to produce the right non-verbal (NV) signals, low rewardingness, lack of certain social skills, etc.

Social competence is easier to define and agree upon in the case of professional social skills: an effective therapist cures more patients, an effective teacher teaches better, an effective salesgirl sells more.

For everyday social skills it is more difficult to give the criteria of success; lack of competence is easier to spot − failure to make friends, or opposite-sex friends, quarrelling and failing to sustain co-operative relationships, finding a number of situations difficult or a source of anxiety and so on.

Self-report methods of assessment

The assessment of social competence is usually based at least in part on some kind of interview or questionnaire. It is generally recognized, however, that self-report measures are far from satisfactory in this field, and need to be used with caution. Behavioural measures are better, but much more difficult to obtain.

Interview Clients for SST are usually assessed by a kind of clinical interview. A neurotic patient with interpersonal problems will probably speak first about his own depression or anxiety, or about the difficult behaviour of others. He can be asked to describe in detail the behaviour which occurs in his main social encounters and relationships, especially the ones which he finds difficult. The interviewer tries to obtain as detailed an account as possible of what happens in these difficult situations, in particular what the patient himself does or fails to do. This can be supplemented by the use of rating scales, on which he reports which situations are most difficult.

Rating scales and questionnaires There are several questionnaires which assess general assertiveness, e.g. the Rathus Assertive Schedule (Rathus 1973). However, since the discovery that individual assertiveness varies greatly between situations, scales have been devised which ask about assertiveness in specific situations. Such scales have been found to correlate with ratings of assertive behaviour ($r = 0.6-0.8$). Other scales have been constructed for measuring social anxiety, and a number of separate factors have been found, as will be described below. Trower, *et al.* (1978) devised a list of thirty situations, on which subjects rate five levels of difficulty, the fifth point being 'avoidance if possible'. Another kind of scale presents a series of difficult situations, and the open-ended responses are then rated or classified by judges.

Self-monitoring This has been developed in connection with behavioural self-control techniques of therapy. The trainee reports systematically on selected aspects of his behaviour and keeps a record of some kind; the behaviour recorded is itself the target of therapy, and this method leads to direct attempts to change the behaviour; in addition the very act of recording is 'reactive', i.e. changes the level of smoking, eating or whatever is being recorded. Social behaviour has rarely been recorded in this way, apart from frequency of dating, and may be more difficult to record accurately. Eisler (1976) suggests that trainees be trained during role playing to record the required aspects of their behaviour. However, self-reports do not always correlate highly with behavioural measures, or with physiological measures of anxiety. Self-reports correlate better with behavioural measures if the self-report inventory describes in detail the situations in which behaviour was observed.

Observation of social performance

Samples of an individual's performance may be obtained and analysed from role playing, or from real life.

Role played   The subject may be presented with several assertiveness situations (e.g. laundry loses shirt), dating situations, or other situations like those in his real environment. Because of the extent of situational variability, it is desirable to sample a number of different kinds of assertiveness situation, or whatever dimension of behaviour is being assessed. We have used a social interaction test based on different phases of a getting-acquainted encounter, with two partners, one male, one female; there are periods of interruption, of non-response and of assertive behaviour. The role playing is videotaped, and scored in terms of the use of elements of verbal behaviour (use of questions, etc.), and NV behaviour (use of facial expressions, etc.) and also in terms of general dimensions of behaviour (e.g. assertiveness, warmth, etc.). Raters are found to have a reasonable degree of agreement on such ratings of behaviour, and indeed on overall judgments of social competence (Trower, *et al.* 1978). While some of these ratings are based on carefully defined criteria, others are deliberately 'subjective', leaving the observer to decide how far the trainee's behaviour is 'warm', 'rewarding', 'socially competent', etc. (Eisler 1976).

   Some doubt has been cast on the validity of role playing by a number of studies in which role-playing performance was compared with performance in staged real-life situations including assertiveness. Bellack, *et al.* (1979) found rather low correlations for male subjects and on certain measures − questions and amount of speech. All that can be said is that the validity of role playing will be greater if a sample of situations is used which are similar to the criterion situation.

Staged events   If a person knows that his assertiveness, for example, is being assessed, his behaviour changes a lot, thereby making the measure invalid. To avoid this happening, in some follow-up studies of assertiveness training events have been created in which, for example, a trainee encounters a person in a waiting room who looks like another trainee, and who makes a series of unreasonable demands for loan of books, notes, etc., the whole encounter being recorded (Rich and Schroeder 1976). This is possibly an unethical procedure but does provide a valid measure of assertiveness.

Observation in real life Several investigators have made use of ratings by colleagues, relations or friends. For example, in some studies of marital therapy each partner has recorded the other's rewarding and unrewarding behaviour for a two-week period (Wills, *et al.* 1974). King, *et al.* (1977), in a multiple-baseline study with a psychotic patient, assessed progress by a therapist unobtrusively accompanying the patient into three situations − a shop, a petrol station and a restaurant. In each situation the patient was asked to make ten requests, and a score was kept of how many he carried out.

Physiological measures

These have been used, for example, in training to reduce public-speaking anxiety (Paul 1966), and heart rate has been used to separate socially anxious and non-anxious groups. However, physiological measures of anxiety have not been found to correlate at all well with self-reported discomfort or with behavioural measures. This is probably because the same state of physiological arousal may sometimes be labelled as euphoria or excitement, and sometimes as anxiety. Some people can perform very effectively while in a state of high physiological arousal, as in the case of many entertainers (Eisler 1976).

The extent and nature of social inadequacy in different groups

The normal population

There is no doubt, from common experience and various social surveys, that a number of kinds of social difficulty are very common: anxiety in various situations, assertiveness problems, difficulty in making friends and in forming relationships with the opposite sex. It is, however, difficult to decide on a cut-off point beyond which a person is said to suffer from social behaviour problems. Possible criteria are: (1) seeking SST, or accepting it when it is available — though this will depend on how readily available it is and how attractively presented; (2) reporting avoidance of everyday situations, or 'great difficulty', etc., or reporting that loneliness, social anxiety, etc. is one of their greatest problems; or (3) behavioural evidence of social inadequacy, such as not having any friends, being very unsuccessful as a salesman, teacher, etc., or the object of complaints from others.

Bryant and Trower (1974) surveyed a 10 per cent sample of Oxford undergraduates and found that a high proportion reported moderate or severe difficulty with common social situations, especially 'approaching others' (36 per cent), 'going to dances/discotheques' (35 per cent) and 'going to parties' (26 per cent). These were the figures for second-year students; first-year students reported much higher levels of difficulty. Nine per cent of second-year students reported 'moderate difficulty' or avoidance of six common situations out of thirty and were regarded as suffering from serious social problems. Zimbardo (1977) surveyed large samples of American and other students aged 18–21 and found that about 40 per cent considered themselves to be 'shy' now, while very few said that they had never been shy. However, the proportion of adults with this problem is probably lower. The results of these and various other surveys suggest that at least 7 per cent of the normal adult population have fairly serious difficulties with social behaviour.

Schizophrenics

They suffer from every possible kind of social skill deficit. Some of these are common to several kinds of patient — poor expression and reception of NV signs (especially face, gesture and posture), low rewardingness, social anxiety and inability to take the role of the other. Other social deficits are more distinctive of schizophrenia — withdrawal from social relationships, inability to conduct sensible conversation, often including poor synchronizing of utterances, very poor self-presentation, e.g. little concern with appearance, and almost total lack of normal social skills. They may also lack such everyday skills as washing and dressing. The fundamental cause of these failures may lie in the cognitive or physiological spheres, and it may be a mistake to look for social processes as causes of schizophrenia, or as useful targets for treatment. SST can modify NV communication without greatly affecting general symptomatology, for example (p. 177). On the other hand, since schizophrenia is evidently partly due to environmental experiences it may be worth looking for social processes behind the symptoms. Possible candidates are absence of relevant personal constructs (Bannister and Salmon 1966) and persistent rule-breaking (Braginsky *et al.* 1969). Another possibility is failure to grasp the essential features of situations − which happens to all of us in some situations − and consequent ability to take part in sensible sequences of behaviour.

Depressives

These also share a number of deficits with other patients, but they also show distinctive forms of failure. Libet and Lewinsohn (1973) developed a category scheme for comparing the social interaction of depressives and controls; they found that the depressed patients had a very low level of verbal activity, low rate of initiation (i.e. they are passive), slow speed of response, and low level of rewardingness. They are also low in self-confidence, feel guilty and depressed, and behave in a 'helpless' manner. Depressives speak in a low pitch and at a slow speed; other aspects of NV communication are also affected − such as their downward gaze and drooping posture. The fundamental process behind these symptoms may be primarily one of mood, but social processes have also been suggested. Lewinsohn (1975) and his collaborators have argued that depressives' lack of social skill leads to their receiving very little positive reinforcement from others, and this produces their depressed state. Seligman (1975) suggested that experience of inability to control events, especially social events, leads to a state of learned helplessness. However, Phillips (1978), in a factorial study, found four types of depressives, as defined by Minnesota Multiphase Personality Inventory (MMPI) scores and social behaviour: two types showed clear social skill deficits, one introverted and the other alienated; the third type had better skills, though of a self-centred and non-sharing kind; and the fourth type had normal skills. Howes and Hokanson (1979) found that subjects who met role-played depressives for seven minutes rejected these people and spoke to them less, but gave expressions of support as they did to role players of physical illness. Depression appeared to elicit a double message of non-genuine reassurance; depressive behaviour was partly instrumental in that it did elicit sympathy.

Neurotics

Many neurotics do not suffer from social skill deficits, although their phobias or other peculiarities may make social life difficult for them. Bryant, *et al.* (1976) found that 28 per cent of a sample of neurotic outpatients were regarded as socially unskilled by clinical psychologists and psychiatrists. They were low in components of both control (assertiveness) and rewardingness, and were deficient in basic skills like conducting conversations. The socially inadequate appeared colder, less assertive, less happy, less controlling, less rewarding and more anxious than the socially adequate group. They were also significantly more likely to have had a history of solitariness, difficulty in making friends and of unsuccessful attempts at 'dating' in adolescence. In terms of elements of behaviour, they tended towards the 'inactive' or unassertive side, being on the whole rather silent, showing little interest in others, speaking very briefly and in a slow and rather monotonous voice, rarely handing over the conversation, sitting very still and rigid, and with a dull, fixed expression. Trower (1980) found that the behaviour which discriminated best between neurotics rated as socially inadequate and other neurotics was their low amount of speech, followed by their low amounts of looking, smiling, gesturing and posture shifting.

Neurotics are often socially isolated. Henderson, *et al.* (1978) found that they had far fewer friends than comparable non-neurotics. Lack of friends is one of the commonest complaints on the part of those seeking SST. This may be due to a low level of rewardingness, which in turn may be due to egocentricity. Another factor is probably inability to emit positive NV signals. Lack of heterosexual contacts is also common among neurotics. This may be lack of contact with the opposite sex ('minimal dating'), or anxiety in the presence of the opposite sex ('heterosexual anxiety'), and these are alternate targets for social skills training. This problem can be assessed by self-rating scales on, for example, the level of anxiety, discomfort or difficulty experienced when asking someone for a date, or going on a first date with someone. The origins of this condition have been suggested to be lack of social skills, conditioned anxiety, or inaccurate perception of own performance together with anticipation of aversive consequences (Curran

1977). Twentyman and McFall (1975) found that after SST a number of shy males showed lower physiologically-measured anxiety while dating.

Neurotics often suffer acutely from social anxiety in a range of social situations. Social anxiety as a trait is the tendency to be made anxious by social situations. Anxiety is produced when people perceive the situation as threatening; there is a state of autonomic arousal, and they label their state of arousal as anxiety, rather than, for example, excitement or eager anticipation (Schachter 1964). A state of social anxiety is produced when people high in interpersonal anxiety are confronted by threatening social situations, but not by physical danger (Endler and Magnusson 1976). Paul (1966), in his study of public-speaking anxiety, obtained ratings on twenty items, such as 'knees tremble', 'moistens lips', 'perspires', etc. The behaviour which is now known to reflect social anxiety includes: breathy voice, rapid speech with speech errors, low level of gaze, tense, flushed and perspiring face, tense and defensive posture and self-touching gestures (Argyle 1975).

Social anxiety can be divided up into smaller factors corresponding to different kinds of social threat. The factors most commonly obtained are:

(1) Fear of performing in public, being the focus of attention.
(2) Fear of conflict, rejection or disapproval.
(3) Fear of intimacy, heterosexual or otherwise.

Other factors which have been obtained are:

(4) Fear of meeting strangers.
(5) Anxiety about assertiveness.
(Stratton and Moore 1977, Richardson and Tasto 1976, Hodges and Felling 1970).

One important behaviour manifestation of social anxiety is avoidance of situations: Bryant and Trower (1974) found that a proportion of a sample of students did not go to parties, pubs or other situations they couldn't cope with.

Social anxiety does correlate (negatively) with assertiveness, but the correlation is about −0.2 to −0.4, so these two forms of failure are fairly independent of one another (Hollandsworth 1976). Social anxiety probably results from negative experiences in the past in certain social situations − leading to anticipation of rejection, etc. in the future. This in turn may be due to lack of social skills in these situations. If so it would be expected that SST would first lead to improved performance, and, a little later, to improved self-reports. Marshall, *et al.* (1977) found that SST improved rated behaviour more than systematic desensitization (SD) did, but that SD had more effect on self-reports of anxiety.

A distinction can be drawn between those patients who have social phobias and those who have inadequate social skills, though the two groups overlap. Since SST produces considerable improvement in neurotics, social deficits may be a basic cause of other symptoms for some of them. On the other hand, the fact that relaxation and desensitization also improve social behaviour suggests that anxiety is simply suppressing skills which are there. Trower, *et al.* (1978) found that socially unskilled patients were helped more by SST than by desensitization; phobics were helped equally by both methods of treatment.

The basic cause of all these problems may be certain specifically neurotic styles of social behaviour. Neurotics are often very unrewarding and fail to send positive NV signals; they are often highly egocentric, in that they have no real interest in other people or their point of view. Neurotics may be unduly hostile, leading to those destructive 'games' intended to put other people down which Berne (1966) described. They have difficulty in accepting the rules of social situations and may engage in sudden demands for intimacy, and other startling forms of behaviour. Hysterics and hypochondriacs engage in narrow ranges of social performance which are sustained because they elicit a certain amount of sympathetic and rewarding response from others (Phillips 1979). Trower (1980) observed that a number of patients engage in a 'self-fulfilling prophecy' in which they engage in behaviour which results in confirming their worst fears about the attitude of others towards them. They may have an excessive desire to be the centre of attention, and engage in inappropriate attention-getting devices.

Alcoholics

Alcoholics have been found to be deficient in social skills. They are poor in everyday skills such as conversation, awkward with others, lonely, socially anxious and low in self-esteem. They are, however, over- rather than underassertive. There is clinical evidence that alcoholics find social situations stressful because of their poor social skills and that they drink to reduce their anxiety, or perhaps to be able to use uninhibited styles of behaviour (van Hasselt, *et al.* 1978).

Delinquents and prisoners

Delinquents have generally been found to be low in various aspects of social skills; they are low in internal locus of control, and this is particularly true of aggressive and sexual offenders. Delinquents have been found to be low in ability to cope with many everyday situations; they behave in a more aggressive and inappropriately assertive manner than controls (Freedman, *et al.* 1978). There is some evidence for lack of perceptual sensitivity (McDavid and Schroder 1957); this can lead them into trouble if they fail to realize how they are annoying other people, so that they get into fights. Most delinquents are hostile towards and unable to relate to people in authority. Sexual offenders are believed to be deficient in heterosexual skills, and these are often the target for treatment. Psychopaths possess certain manipulative skills but are lacking in empathy — ability to see another's point of view, and concern for the welfare of others.

However, within any group of offenders there may be a range of social skill deficits. Henderson (unpublished report), in a study of 107 aggressive offenders, found several distinct sub-groups: (1) psychiatrically disturbed and hostile (bad relations and aggressive within family); (2) extroverted and hostile; (3) inhibited (few friends and poor relations with groups); and (4) controlled (psychiatrically normal but with a high rate of unemployment).

Disturbed children

The social behaviour of children can probably fail in as many ways as that of adults. However, two particular types of failure have been singled out most often for SST — aggression and withdrawal. Aggressiveness is a quite common form of disturbance, especially in overactive boys. Withdrawal, as measured by unpopularity or infrequent interaction, is partly associated with low assertiveness. However, it may also be due to lack of other social skills such as rewardingness and ability to sustain everyday social encounters (van Hasselt *et al.* 1979).

Components of socially skilled performance, and how they can fail

Skills, plans and feedback in skilled performance

Competent social performance is similar to performance of a motor skill (p. 2). This analogy emphasizes the motivation, goals and plans of interactors. It is postulated that every interactor is trying to achieve some goal, whether he is aware of it or not. It also emphasizes the importance of feedback processes: interactors, like performers of motor skills, continually modify their behaviour in response to its effects.

The skill system may go wrong in a number of ways. Many patients are passive and dependent, lacking in persistence, self-control and self-direction. They take the subordinate side of encounters and leave other people to take all the initiative. Some individuals are very unresponsive to feedback, either because they don't notice the effect their behaviour has on others, or because they don't know what corrective action to take. Snyder (1974) found that individuals vary in the extent to which they monitor their own social performance and he devised a scale for assessing this aspect of social competence. The plans may be inappropriate, as in the case of Berne's patients who wanted to make other people feel uncomfortable or look foolish (Berne 1966).

Reinforcement

One effect of reinforcement is in the control of others' behaviour. If A consistently gives small signs of approval immediately after B produces some form of behaviour, the frequency of that behaviour is rapidly increased (or decreased following disapproval). This is one of the main processes whereby people are able to modify each other's behaviour in the desired direction. Clearly, if people do not give clear, immediate and consistent reinforcements, positive and negative, they will not be able to influence others in this way, and social encounters will be correspondingly more frustrating and difficult for them. This appears to be a common problem with many psychiatric patients, who characteristically fail to control or try to over-control others.

Rewardingness also affects popularity. There are a number of different sources of popularity and unpopularity but there is little doubt that being a source of rewards is one of the most important (Rubin 1973). A person may be rewarding because the interaction with him is enjoyable, e.g. making love, playing squash; he may be rewarding because he is kind, helpful, interesting, etc.; and people are rewarding just by being attractive or of high status. One of the most common characteristics of socially unskilled patients is their low rewardingness; this is particularly the case with chronic schizophrenics, who have been described as 'socially bankrupt' (Longabaugh, *et al.* 1966).

Verbal communication

Socially inadequate people are usually very ineffective in the sphere of verbal communication. They often speak very little, fail to ask questions or to show an interest in others, to produce the kinds of utterances which will be effective in particular situations or to sustain conversations. They may be inadequate in the use of NV communication to accompany speech. Trower (1980) found that the main difference in behaviour between socially inadequate and other patients was that the latter talked more.

Completing and elaborating verbal utterances   Utterances are accompanied by vocal stress, pitch and timing, by facial expressions and by gestures. These NV signals elaborate utterances in a number of important ways (p. 8). Some socially incompetent people fail to send these signals, with the result that their utterances may be not only uninteresting but also ambiguous, and it may not be clear what kind of answer is expected.

Managing synchronizing   This is accomplished mainly by NV signals, like head-nods, uh-huh noises and shifts of gaze (p. 9). If a person cannot manage these signals, or recognize them in others, there will be interruptions and long silences.

Sending feedback signals   A listener in a conversation usually produces 'listening behaviour': head-nods, glances and grunts to show that he is still attending. More important, he also sends feedback on his reactions to the other's behaviour, whether he agrees or disagrees, is interested or bored, etc. Speakers need this feedback and find it very difficult talking to people who don't give it. Mental patients are often very unresponsive and give the impression of not being interested and of not reacting to what has been said.

Non-verbal communication of interpersonal attitudes and emotions

Several studies have shown that some of the main differences between socially inadequate people and others consists of more smiling, gaze and other NV signals by the latter (p. 10). Attitudes towards others, e.g. friendly or hostile, superior or inferior, are communicated mainly by NV cues (see p. 13). The same is true of emotions. The face is the most important channel for these messages, followed by tone of voice, though posture, gestures and gaze also convey this kind of information. This is a sphere in which social performance often fails: if interactors do not send clear facial and vocal signals, others simply do not know what the performer's attitudes or feelings are. The most common form of failure is where face and voice are simply devoid of expression. Another kind of failure is where the attitudes communicated are mainly negative (e.g. sarcastic, suspicious, aloof), and the emotions likewise (depressed, angry, etc.).

Perception

If we are going to respond effectively to another person, he or she must be perceived accurately. There are great individual differences in possession of appropriate personal constructs, and in accuracy of impression formation. On the other hand, research has not found a clear relationship between perceptual accuracy and social competence. Research suggests that it is important to be sensitive to NV communication and to have a complex set of categories for forming impressions of people, but most important to empathize with others. It is undesirable to be oversensitive, for example, to cues of rejection.

Mental patients and people with inadequate social skills are often deficient in person perception. We have found that socially unskilled neurotics often do not attend to or show much interest in other people, and may not look very much (Trower, *et al.* 1978). Young (1979) found that neurotics were more sensitive than other people to cues of rejection. However, it is possible for people to make their initially inaccurate perceptions come true; if A thinks that B dislikes him he can easily make this happen (Trower 1980a). Manic and paranoid patients are notorious for the inaccuracy of their perception of events, and delinquents have been found to be very insensitive — failing to recognize either approval or annoyance in others (McDavid and Schroder 1957). Beck (1967) interviewed depressive patients and controls and found that the depressives engaged in unrealistic and illogical cognitive distortion; for example, exaggerating their problems, low self-evaluation, ideas of deprivation and self-criticism.

The most accurate social perceivers are people who are well adjusted, intelligent, cognitively complex, not authoritarian, and somewhat introverted and detached (Argyle 1969).

Taking the role of the other

There are individual differences in the ability to see another person's point of view, as measured by tests in which subjects are asked to describe situations as perceived by others. Those who are good at it have been found to do better at a number of social tasks (Feffer and Suchotliff 1966) and to be more altruistic. Meldman (1967) found that psychiatric patients are more egocentric, i.e. talked about themselves more than controls, and it has been our experience that socially unskilled patients have great difficulty in taking the role of the other.

Sequences of interaction

I have discussed earlier the ways in which sequences of conversation and other kinds of interaction are constructed (p. 17). Socially inadequate people often have great difficulty in sustaining conversation, or performing effectively the sequences of moves in particular situations. Hayden, *et al.* (1977) found that emotionally disturbed boys were less able than controls to reorder a set of photos to show an interaction sequence. Here are examples of how sequences can go wrong:

(1) Failure to initiate, the individual only responds to others (mentioned under Skills, plans and feedback).
(2) Failure to hand the conversation over to others:

> A: I went to Swindon yesterday.
> B: Oh yes.
>   (End of conversation.)

A should have added a handing-over phase such as 'I was in Swindon yesterday; have you been there recently?'; or 'I went to Swindon yesterday; an extraordinary thing happened.'

(3) Failure to hand over conversation after answering a question:

> A: Where do you come from?
> B: Swindon.
>   (End of conversation.)

B should have used a double, or 'pro-active' move, of the type 'I come from Swindon; where do *you* come from?'

These features are described in Chapter 1.

Situations, and their component features

A number of studies have shown that patients are *less* variable in their behaviour between situations, and that psychotics are less variable than neurotics (e.g. Moos 1968, Trower 1980b). This means that the patients are failing to respond appropriately to the requirements of different situations. Snyder and Monson (1975) found that subjects high in neuroticism and subjects low in self-monitoring (which correlated at $r = +0.29$) were both insensitive to situational influences. This suggests that training to deal with different situations may be useful. Furthermore, while some people are socially incompetent in many situations, others find only certain situations difficult. To carry out SST for such people it has been necessary to analyse the main features of situations, and to find out where these people are going wrong. Just as a newcomer might be baffled by, say, American football, so a newcomer might be baffled by certain social situations. What does he need to know to be able to perform competently? To understand a new game one needs to know such things as the goals (how to score and win), the moves allowed, the rules, the roles and the physical setting and equipment. Similar information is needed for a social situation: the goals, rules, roles, physical setting, repertoire of moves, concepts used and special skills.

Goals   In all situations there are certain goals which are commonly attainable. It is often fairly obvious what these are, but socially inadequate people may simply not know what parties are for, for example, or may think that the purpose of a selection interview is vocational guidance.

Rules   All situations have rules about what may or may not be done in them. Socially inexperienced people are often ignorant or mistaken about the rules. It would obviously be impossible to play a game without knowing the rules, and the same applies to social situations.

Special skills   Many social situations require special social skills, as in the case of various kinds of public speaking and interviewing, but also in such everyday situations as dates and parties. A person with little experience of a particular situation may find that he lacks the special skills needed for it (see Argyle, *et al.*, in press).

Handling relationships   Many people with social-behaviour problems report difficulties with relationships. One of the most common is difficulty in making friends, which in turn is due to some of the processes already described – low rewardingness, and poor NV communication. Special skills are also required, such as inviting others to appropriate social events, and increasing self-disclosure (p. 23). Assertiveness training has played a central part in much American SST, and the relevant skills are usually taught by British trainers.

Many socially inadequate people have problems with assertiveness, and need to be taught the necessary skills (p. 24). Other kinds of relationships have difficulties which can be understood in terms of the concepts of goals, rules, activities, etc. which provide a map of the difficulties (p. 25).

Self-presentation

A normally competent interactor sends mainly NV signals to indicate his role, status or other aspects of his identity. From these signals others know what to expect, including what rewards are likely to be forthcoming, and how to deal with him. Self-presentation can go wrong in a number of ways: (1) bogus claims which are unmasked; (2) being too 'grey', i.e. sending too little information; (3) sending too much, overdramatizing, as hysterical personalities sometimes do; (4) inappropriate self-presentation, e.g. a bank manager who dresses like a criminal, a female research student who looks and sounds like a retired professor. Several studies have found that mental patients, both male and female, are judged to be less attractive than controls, even before they became ill (p. 28).

Self-disclosure   This is a related process to self-presentation, and is particularly important in getting to know people and in making friends. Self-disclosure should proceed at the right speed, and be matched and reciprocated. Some socially inadequate people produce far too much too soon, while others produce no self-disclosure at all. It has been found that mentally disturbed people engage in less self-disclosure than normals, and this has been regarded as one of the processes responsible for their condition (Chaikin and Derlega 1976).

The effectiveness of social skills training with different kinds of patients

SST with patients has consisted usually of role playing combined with coaching, modelling and video playback in groups. In American studies the focus has often been on assertiveness. Often there has been an emphasis on correcting NV communication. A few programmes have been based on social psychological research into social inter-action and tried to correct some of the other processes described in the last section (Trower, *et al.* 1978). It is becoming common in clinical practice to combine SST for patients with cognitive therapy, such as Rational Emotive Therapy. Although each diagnostic category is associated with different forms of social skill deficits, it is not necessary for SST that a diagnosis be made at all: all that is required is an analysis of the failure of social performance.

Chronic inpatients

A number of studies have been carried out in the USA on schizo-phrenics, depressives and other inpatients. SST has been directed towards increasing assertiveness and improving NV communication. The criteria used have been ratings of behaviour in the hospital, or observations of role playing. Two main designs have been used. Clinical studies have consisted of the intensive training of 1−4 patients over a period of time, comparing performance after the end of treat-ment with performance during a baseline period. In the 'multiple baseline' method, treatment has focused on one behaviour at a time; the baseline for each behaviour is taken during the period before treatment for it started. Clinical studies have the drawback of lacking a control group to allow for the effect of assessment or treatment in general. 'Analogue' designs consist of experimental trials with one or more control groups and before and after measures, but usually a fairly short set of standard training exercises.

All of these studies have obtained positive results, in that the treated patients were more assertive, and used more gaze and other aspects of NV communication (e.g. Goldsmith and McFall 1975, Goldstein 1973). However, there has usually been poor generaliza-tion, e.g. from the assertiveness problems on which patients have been trained to other assertiveness situations. More important, in most studies we do not know whether there would be generalization to situations outside the hospital, since the patients apparently con-tinued to be inpatients, and there is no evidence that their clinical symptoms were much affected. The best results have been obtained in intensive training of 1−4 patients, using a multiple-baseline method and typically 30 hours of training. A number of depressed and schizophrenic patients have been trained up to competent performance in settings inside and outside the hospital, and were discharged (Hersen 1979). Zeiss, *et al.* (1979) found that SST relieved depression as much as cognitive training and training to seek pleasant events, though the effects were not specifically related to the form of treatment. These authors interpret their results in terms of improvement of morale or feelings of personal efficacy rather than social skills.

It should be mentioned that there are two other forms of social treatment for chronic inpatients which have succeeded in improving both social behaviour and clinical condition − milieu therapy and the token economy. Paul and Lentz (1977) found great improvement in chronic schizophrenics over two years of intensive treatment; systematic behaviour reinforcement with a token economy was more effective than milieu therapy.

Zigler and Phillips (1962) distinguished between schizophrenics with good and bad pre-morbid social competence, and their process−reactive distinction has been widely used. Presumably, process schizophrenics did not previously possess adequate social skills, whereas the reactive schizophrenics did.

Neurotic outpatients

Several British and American studies have been carried out on outpatients, using experimental control group designs and a six-months' follow-up. The patients selected for these studies have been neurotics judged to be socially inadequate. The target behaviours have been general social skills, heterosexual skills, assertiveness and verbal and non-verbal behaviour, as well as removal of clinical symptoms. The criterion measures used have included role-played tests but also self- and other-ratings of behaviour in real life. Methods used have included the usual role playing, modelling and coaching, but also more specialized methods based on social psychological analysis. In all studies SST had positive effects on the behaviour of patients, but so did psychotherapy, desensitization and relaxation therapy. Argyle, *et al.* (1974) found that SST did as well as twice as much psychotherapy, and lasted longer. Trower, *et al.* (1978) found that SST led to more improvement of specific social skills, and specifically social anxieties, than did desensitization. Maxwell (unpublished observations) studied the effects of various kinds of training on self-referred clients for SST, who in my experience would mostly be fairly neurotic. SST with video playback was by far the most effective, in terms of self-ratings and ratings of role-played encounters by others. Vitalo (1971) found that SST had more effect on warmth, empathy and genuineness than did traditional group therapy. On the other hand, therapy had more effect on clinical measures.

The results of these follow-up studies are quite different from those for inpatients, in that real-life behaviour was affected and clinical symptoms were reduced. On the other hand, there is no clear evidence that SST is superior to other forms of treatment; its main advantage is in the area of specifically social skills and anxieties. It is very interesting that social competence can evidently be improved by therapies such as desensitization and relaxation. (Reviews of SST for inpatients and outpatients can be found in Hersen and Bellack 1976, Marzillier 1978 and Bellack and Hersen 1979.)

Alcoholics and drug addicts

These two groups have been found to be deficient in social skills (p. 168). SST for alcoholics has been directed at increasing their ability to resist social pressure to drink, and to dealing better with situations which are found stressful and which induce drinking. Drug addicts have been trained in similar ways, and in addition have been trained in some of the basic skills needed in straight society. In both cases it has been recognized that skills in addition to assertiveness are required, especially skills needed to make clients attractive and acceptable to normal people. Follow-up studies have shown that SST is successful in reducing intake of alcohol and drugs, though the effects have not been very long-lasting in some cases. This has led to the inclusion of SST in more comprehensive packages of treatment, including desensitization and cognitive therapy (van Hasselt, *et al.* 1978). Training in problem-solving ability, including finding alternative solutions to difficult social situations, has been used successfully with alcoholics (Intagliata 1978).

Delinquents and prisoners

A number of studies have been carried out on SST with delinquents. The main aims of treatment have been to improve social skills in everyday situations like job interviews, to increase internal control, and to reduce aggressive behaviour. SST with role playing and modelling has been found to be fairly successful, and superior to group discussion in reducing recidivism, improving social skills and reducing aggressiveness. SST has been more successful with delinquents who are anxious or high in internal control (Ollendick and Hersen 1979, Goldstein, *et al.* 1978). SST with adult convicts has been confined mainly to sexual and aggressive offenders. Sexual offenders are taught the social skills of courtship, aggressive offenders the social skills of assertion and persuasion. No controlled studies have been reported, but clinical studies without control groups have obtained positive results (e.g. Crawford and Allen 1977). Pre-release training using role playing and modelling has been used successfully to train prisoners in how to get a job, find accommodation and deal with other problems in the outside world (Sarason and Ganzer 1971). Self-presentation skills are also important: Kurtberg, *et al.* (1968) reduced the recidivism rate by plastic surgery to remove scars and tattooing in a group of heavily disfigured delinquents.

Disturbed children

SST has been given to children who are withdrawn, unpopular and unassertive, and to children who are aggressive and disturbed in other ways. SST with children has grown rapidly during recent years. Children who are unpopular are more likely to be delinquent, mentally disturbed or academically unsuccessful later; and unpopularity is associated with poor social skills, though being physically unattractive, bad at sport, or having the wrong social background are also relevant. Social inadequacy in children can be assessed by parent- or teacher-ratings, or by role-played performance (Rinn and Markle 1979).

Follow-up studies have used the multiple baseline and experimental analogue designs. Criteria used have included sociometric questionnaires to other children and teacher ratings, as well as self-reports and role-play methods. The training methods used have consisted mainly of modelling and coaching; the videotape-recorder has been little used. It has been suggested that more collaboration should be brought about with teachers and parents: Goldstein, *et al.* (1978) trained staff members, peer group leaders and other inmates of an institution to observe, coach, prompt and reward competent skill performance by trainees. Most studies have obtained positive results: trainees became more assertive, less aggressive, more popular, or better conversationalists, in different studies, though few long-term follow-ups have been carried out. The most successful method of training was modelling, and coaching has also been successful.

Shure (1978) has developed methods of training children in 'alternative problem solving', that is to think of different forms of social behaviour to attain ends, in interaction with peers. They are also trained to anticipate the consequences of, for example, grabbing a toy from another and in thinking of others' feelings. Parents can help their children to acquire these skills by a certain kind of dialogue. This form of training has been found to lead to improved behaviour and social skills at school.

SST with disturbed adolescents has focused on the skills of dealing with the peer group and dating, of dealing with parents and other people in authority and the skills of obtaining and keeping jobs (Trower 1978). Most adults who are socially inadequate also had problems during adolescence and particular skills are required during adolescence. The methods which have been most successful with this age group include training in taking the role of the other (Chandler 1973) as well as the usual methods. Some therapists have used a multiple-baseline design while others have used more general role-playing procedures covering the skills needed by adolescents (Lindsay, *et al.* 1979). Other schemes have been designed for normal adolescents: Haynes and Avery (1979) succeeded in improving self-disclosure and empathy skills.

Normal people with social difficulties: assertiveness training

This is one of the most widely-practised forms of SST. Assertiveness is taken to include a number of somewhat different but, it is believed, related patterns of social behaviour. In the early days of behaviour therapy this treatment was devised for people who were too passive and submissive. Assertiveness is now taken to include the ability to say no, the ability to ask for favours or to make requests and the ability to express positive and negative feelings (Lazarus 1973). It is also often taken to include an individual's ability to stand up for his rights, and to act in his own best interests. Positive assertiveness — expressing affection or approval — is distinguished from negative assertiveness — expressing disagreement, making protests, etc. Another aspect is simply taking the initiative in social behaviour. Assertiveness training has focused on the negative side of assertiveness, such as disagreement, rather than on the positive side, such as expressing positive feelings (Griffiths 1979). Typical instances of assertiveness are dealing with laundries who lose shirts and with other students who borrow notes and fail to return them. It was originally believed that assertiveness was a general trait; however a number of studies have shown that assertiveness consists of several different factors, corresponding to different situations, and different modes of response (e.g. Eisler, *et al.* 1975). The most valid measures of assertiveness ask for self-reports for a number of specific assertiveness situations (p. 161).

It is believed in some quarters that assertiveness is the whole of social skills. However, research in social psychology has repeatedly shown that there are two main dimensions of social performance: control (or assertiveness) and warmth (or concern with social relationships). Making friends, of either sex, is not a matter of bullying the others to be friendly, but requires quite different skills. Assertiveness includes those social skills which are intended to obtain rewards for the performer but at the risk of losing social rewards, hence the fear of rejection and the link with social anxiety. Controlling skills use verbal behaviour − directing, ordering, persuading − and NV behaviour − loud and firm tone of voice, unsmiling face, erect but relaxed posture, breaking gaze last (Argyle 1975). However, assertiveness alone is not likely to be successful unless accompanied by sufficient rewards. Control is more successful when it is not authoritarian: when the controller advises, persuades, co-ordinates, explains and suggests rather than orders or criticizes. And assertive behaviour should be distinguished from aggressive behaviour (Rich and Schroeder 1976).

Heterosexual skills

The condition may be defined as lack of contact with the opposite sex ('minimal dating'), or anxiety in the presence of the opposite sex ('heterosexual anxiety'), and these are alternate targets for SST. It can be assessed by self-rating scales on, for example, the level of anxiety, discomfort or difficulty experienced when asking someone for a date, or going on a first date.

Social skills are not the only source of heterosexual success, however. Others include physical attractiveness, low heterosexual anxiety and positive self-evaluation. All have been shown to be important and it is clear that attractiveness is important for females; some trainers advise their clients in how to improve this. Glasgow and Arkowitz (1975) found that social skills were important for females but that low-dating males suffered more from negative self-evaluation. What produces heterosexual success? There is rather inconsistent evidence that successful males initiate more, talk more, respond verbally to appropriate cues, and can adjust better to negative reactions.

Heterosexual anxiety can be reduced and frequency of dates increased by a number of anxiety-reduction methods. One quite successful form of anxiety-reduction therapy has been 'practice dating'; trainees have six dates arranged with other trainees (Arkowitz 1977). Heterosexual anxiety can also be treated by desensitization, and this too has been quite successful (Galassi and Galassi 1979).

When SST has been compared with other methods of anxiety reduction, it has usually been more successful, e.g. in frequency of dating, self-ratings and other-ratings of skill or anxiety. The methods used have included video playback and homework, and the coaching and role playing has been directed to the specific social skills required at different stages of dating and different situations.

Conclusions

Studies of the social behaviour of mental patients have discovered that many of them suffer from social skills deficits. The social behaviour of schizophrenics is inadequate in many ways but this may not be the cause of other symptoms. The poor social skills of depressives may result in their receiving little reinforcement from others, which in turn produces their depressed condition. About a third of neurotics are socially incompetent, suffering from social anxiety, low assertiveness, and inability to make friends. Alcoholics are also very poor in everyday social skills, though they are not lacking in assertiveness. Delinquents and prisoners suffer from a variety of social deficits, including lack of everyday social skills, which leads them to behave in an unduly aggressive way: some are lacking in perceptual sensitivity and empathy. An important development has been the sub-division of familiar clinical groups into smaller groups, with distinctive social behaviour problems. The most common deficits in children are aggressiveness and withdrawal. There are a variety of different forms of social skill deficits, many of which cannot be explained by lack of assertiveness.

The most successful methods of SST are role playing combined with coaching, modelling, videotape-recording playback and homework, conducted in groups. More specialized methods have been developed for tackling particular deficits, based on the social–psychological understanding of the processes used.

SST is being used for a wide variety of patients. For chronic inpatients it has been found successful in improving assertiveness and NV communication within the hospital, and with intensive training over a period of 30 hours performance may be improved in other settings. For neurotic outpatients their social behaviour in real life is greatly improved, and clinical symptoms are reduced. However, SST is not much better than other forms of treatment, though it does have more effect on specifically social difficulties and anxieties. Success has been reported with alcoholics and drug addicts, though the results have not always been long-lasting. SST with delinquents and prisoners has succeeded in reducing aggressiveness, improving heterosexual skills, and in improving their ability to deal with everyday life. Withdrawn and aggressive children have also been helped by means of SST. Normal people with social difficulties can be greatly helped, especially by assertiveness training and training in heterosexual skills. However, within each of these categories there is a wide range of individual differences in the nature of the social inadequacy.

I believe that the way ahead in this sphere is more research into the specific deficits of particular clinical groups, and the use of special training techniques based on an analysis of the processes used. Examples are perceptual skills training, use of situational analysis for people who can't cope with particular situations, and sequence analysis for people who can't conduct conversations (see p. 202).

References

Argyle, M. (1969). *Social Interaction*. London: Methuen.
_____ (1975). *Bodily Communication*. London: Methuen.
Argyle, M., Bryant, B. and Trower, P. (1974). Social skills training and psychotherapy: a comparative study. *Psychol. Med.* 4, 435–43.
Argyle, M., Furnham, A. and Graham, J. A. (1981). *Social Situations*. Cambridge University Press.
Arkowitz, H. (1977). Measurement and modification of minimal dating behavior. *In* Hersen, M. (ed.). *Progress in Behavior Modification*. New York: Academic Press, vol. 5.
Bannister, D. and Salmon, P. (1966). Schizophrenic thought disorder: specific or diffuse? *Br. J. Med. Psychol.* 39, 215–19.
Beck, A. T. (1967). *Depression: Clinical, Experimental and Theoretical Aspects*. New York: Harper and Row.
Bellack, A. S. and Hersen, M. (eds) (1979). *Research and Practice in Social Skills Training*. New York and London: Plenum.

Bellack, A. S., Hersen, M. and Lamparski, D. (1979). Role-play tests for assessing social skills: are they valid? Are they useful? *J. Consult. Clin. Psychol.* 47, 335–42.

Berne, E. (1966). *Games People Play*. London: Deutsch.

Braginsky, B. M., Braginsky, D. D. and Ring, K. (1969). *Methods of Madness. The Mental Hospital as a Last Resort*. New York: Holt, Rinehart and Winston.

Bryant, B. and Trower, P. (1974). Social difficulty in a student population. *Br. J. Educ. Psychol.* 44, 13–21.

Bryant, B., Trower, P., Yardley, K., Urbieta, H. and Letemendia, F. (1976). A survey of social inadequacy among psychiatric outpatients. *Psychol. Med.* 6, 101–12.

Chaikin, A. L. and Derlega, V. J. (1976). Self-disclosure. *In* Thibaut, J. W., Spence, J. T. and Carson, R. C. (eds). *Contemporary Topics in Social Psychology*. Morristown, N.J.: General Learning Press, pp. 177–210.

Chandler, M. J. (1973). Egocentrism and anti-social behavior: the assessment and training of social perspective-taking skills. *Dev. Psychol.* 9, 326–32.

Crawford, D. and Allen, J. (1977). *A Social Skills Training Program with Sex Offenders*. Presented at the International Conference on Love and Attraction, Swansea.

Curran, J. P. (1977). Skills training as an approach to the treatment of heterosexual-social anxiety. *Psychol. Bull.* 84, 140–57.

Eisler, R. M. (1976). The behavioral assessment of social skills. *In* Hersen, M. and Bellack, A. S. (eds). *Behavioral Assessment: A Practical Handbook*. New York: Pergamon Press, pp. 369–95.

Eisler, R. M., Hersen, M., Miller, P. M. and Blanchard, E. B. (1975). Situational determinants of assertive behavior. *J. Consult. Clin. Psychol.* 43, 330–40.

Endler, N. S. and Magnusson, D. (1976). *Interactional Psychology and Personality*. Washington: Hemisphere.

Feffer, M. and Suchotliff, L. (1966). Decentering implications of social interactions. *J. Pers. Soc. Psychol.* 4, 415–22.

Freedman, B. J., Rosenthal, L., Donahoe, C. P., Schlundt, D. G. and McFall, R. M. (1978). A social-behavioral analysis of skill deficits in delinquent and non-delinquent adolescent boys. *J. Consult. Clin. Psychol.* 46, 1448–62.

Galassi, J. and Galassi, M. (1979). A comparison of the factor structure of an assertion scale across sex and population. *Behav. Ther.* 10, 117–28.

Glasgow, R. E. and Arkowitz, H. (1975). The behavioral assessment of male and female social competence in dyadic heterosexual interaction. *Behav. Ther.* 6, 488–95.

Goldsmith, J. B. and McFall, R. M. (1975). Development and evaluation of an interpersonal skill-training programme for psychiatric in-patients. *J. Abnorm. Psychol.* 84, 57–8.

Goldstein, A. P. (1973). *Structured Learning Therapy: Toward a Psychotherapy for the Poor*. New York: Academic Press.

Goldstein, A. P. *et al.* (1978). Training aggressive delinquents in prosocial behavior. *J. Youth Adol.* 7, 73–92.

Griffiths, R. D. P. (1979). Social skills and psychological disorder. *In* Singleton, W. T., Spurgeon, P. and Stammers, R. B. (eds). *The Analysis of Social Skill*. New York and London: Plenum, 39–78.

van Hasselt, V. B., Hersen, M. and Milliones, J. (1978). Social skills training for alcoholics and drug addicts; a review. *Add. Behav.* 3, 221–33.

van Hasselt, V. B., Hersen, M., Whitehill, M. B. and Bellack, S. C. (1979). Social skill assessment and training for children: an evaluative review. *Behav. Res. Ther.* 17, 413–37.

Hayden, B. *et al.* (1977). Interpersonal conceptual structures, predictive accuracy, and social adjustment of emotionally disturbed boys. *J. Abnorm. Psychol.* 86, 315–20.

Haynes, L. A. and Avery, A. W. (1979). Training adolescents in self-disclosure and empathy skills. *J. Consult. Psychol.* 20, 526–30.

Henderson, S., Duncan-Jones, P., McAuley, H. and Ritchie, K. (1978). The patient's primary group. *Br. J. Psychiat.* 132, 74–86.

Hersen, M. (1979). Modification of skill deficits in psychiatric patients. *In* Bellack, A. S. and Hersen, M. (eds). *Research and Practice in Social Skills Training*. New York and London: Plenum, 189–236.

Hodges, W. F. and Felling, J. P. (1970). Types of stressful situations and their relation to trait anxiety and sex. *J. Consult. Clin. Psychol.* 34, 333–7.

Hollandsworth, J. G. (1976). Further investigation of the relationship between expressed fear and assertiveness. *Behav. Res. Ther.* 12, 1–8.

Howes, M. J. and Hokanson, J. E. (1979). Conversational and social responses to depressive interpersonal behavior. *J. Abnorm. Psychol.* 88, 625–34.

Intagliata, J. C. (1978). Increasing the interpersonal problem-solving skills of an alcoholic population. *J. Consult. Clin. Psychol.* 46, 489–98.

King, L. W., Liberman, R. P., Roberts, J. and Bryan, F. (1977). Personal effectiveness: a structured therapy for improving social and emotional skills. *Eur. J. Behav. Anal. Mod.* 2, 82–9.

Kurtberg, R. L., Safar, H. and Cavior, N. (1968). Surgical and social rehabilitation of adult offenders. *In Proceedings of the 76th Annual Convention of the American Psychological Association*, vol. 3, pp. 649–50.

Lazarus, A. A. (1973). On assertive behavior: a brief note. *Behav. Ther.* 4, 697–9.

Lewinsohn, P. M. (1975). The behavioral study and treatment of depression. *In* Hersen, M., Eisler, R. M. and Miller, P. M. (eds). *Progress in Behavior Modification*. New York: Academic Press, vol. 1.

Libet, J. M. and Lewinsohn, P. M. (1973). Concept of social skills with special reference to the behavior of depressed persons. *J. Consult. Clin. Psychol.* 40, 304–12.

Lindsay, W. R., Symons, R. S. and Sweet, T. (1979). A programme for teaching social skills to socially inept adolescents: description and evaluation. *J. Adol.* 2, 215–25.

Longabaugh, R., Eldred, S. H., Bell, N. W. and Sherman, L. J. (1966). The interactional world of the chronic schizophrenic patient. *Psychiatry* 29, 319–44.

McDavid, J., and Schroder, H. M. (1957). The interpretation of approval and disapproval by delinquent and non-delinquent adolescents. *J. Pers.* 25. 539–49.

Marshall, W. C., Stoian, M. and Andrews, W. R. (1977). Skills training and self-administered desensitization in the reduction of public speaking anxiety. *Behav. Res. Ther.* 15, 115–17.

Marzillier, J. (1978). Outcome studies of skills training: a review. *In* Trower, P., Bryant, B. and Argyle, M. (eds). *Social Skills and Mental Health*. London: Methuen.

Meldman, M. J. (1967). Verbal behavior analysis of self-hyperattentionism. *Dis. Nerv. Syst.* 28, 469–73.

Moos, R. (1968). Situational analysis of a therapeutic community milieu. *J. Abnorm. Psychol.* 73, 49–61.

Ollendick, T. H. and Hersen, M. (1979). Social skills training for juvenile delinquents. *Behav. Res. Ther.* 17, 547–54.

Paul, G. L. (1966). *Insight vs. Desensitization in Psychotherapy*. Stanford University Press.

Paul, G. L. and Lentz, R. J. (1977). *Psychosocial Treatment of Chronic Mental Patients*. Cambridge, Mass.: Harvard University Press.

Phillips, E. L. (1978). *The Social Skills Basis of Psychopathology*. New York: Grune and Stratton.

Phillips, E. L. (1979). Social skills instruction as adjunctive/alternative to psychotherapy. *In* Singleton, W. T., Spurgeon, P. and Stammers, R. B. (eds). *The Analysis of Social Skill*. New York and London: Plenum, pp. 159–74.

Rathus, S. A. (1973). A 30-item schedule for assessing assertive behavior. *Behav. Ther.* 4, 398–406.

Rich, A. R. and Schroeder, H. E. (1976). Research issues in assertiveness training. *Psychol. Bull.* 83, 1081–96.

Richardson, F. C. and Tasto, D. L. (1976). Development and factor analysis of a social anxiety inventory. *Behav. Ther.* 7, 453–62.

Rinn, R. C. and Markle, A. (1979). Modification of social skill deficits in children. *In* Bellack, A. S. and Hersen, M. (eds). *Research and Practice in Social Skills Training*. New York and London: Plenum, 107–29.

Rubin, Z. (1973). *Liking and Loving*. New York: Holt, Rinehart and Winston.

Sarason, I. G. and Ganzer, V. J. (1971). *Modeling: an Approach to the Rehabilitation of Juvenile Offenders*. Baltimore, M.D.: U.S. Departments of Health, Education and Welfare.

Schachter, S. (1964). The interaction of cognitive and physiological determinants of emotional state. *Advances in Experimental Social Psychology*. vol. 1, pp. 49–80.

Seligman, M. E. P. (1975). *Helplessness*. San Francisco: Freeman.

Shure, M. B. (1978). *Problem-Solving Techniques in Child-Rearing*. San Francisco: Jossey-Bass.

Snyder, M. (1974). Self-monitoring of expressive behavior. *J. Pers. Soc. Psychol.* 30, 526–37.

Snyder, M. and Monson, T. C. (1975). Persons, situations, and the control of social behavior. *J. Pers. Soc. Psychol.* 32, 637–44.

Stratton, T. T. and Moore, C. L. (1977). Application of the robust factor concept to the fear survey schedule. *J. Behav. Ther. Exp. Psychiat.* 8, 229–35.

Trower, P. (1978). Skills training for adolescents: a viable treatment alternative? *J. Add.* 1, 319–29.

—— (1980). How to lose friends and influence nobody: an analysis of social failure. *In* Singleton, W. T., Spurgeon, P. and Stammers, R. B. (eds). *The Analysis of Social Skill.* New York and London: Plenum, pp. 257–73.

—— (1980). Situational analysis of the components and processes of socially skilled and unskilled patients. *J. Consult. Clin. Psychol.* 48, 327–39.

—— (1981). Social Skill Disorder: Mechanisms of Failure. *In* Gilmour, R. and Duck, S. (eds). *Personal Relationships in Disorder.* London: Academic Press.

Trower, P., Bryant, B. and Argyle, M. (1978). *Social Skills and Mental Health.* London: Methuen.

Trower, P., Yardley, K., Bryant, B. M. and Shaw, P. H. (1978). The treatment of social failure: a comparison of anxiety reduction and skill-acquisition on two social problems. *Behav. Mod.* 2, 41–60.

Twentyman, G. T. and McFall, R. M. (1975). Behavioral training in shy males. *J. Consult. Clin. Psychol.* 43, 384–95.

Vitalo, R. (1971). Teaching improved interpersonal functioning as a preferred mode of treatment. *J. Clin. Psychol.* 22, 166–171.

Wills, T. A., Weiss, R. L. and Patterson, G. R. (1974). A behavioral analysis of the determination of marital satisfaction. *J. Consult. Clin. Psychol.* 42, 802–11.

Young, G. C. D. (1979). *Selective Perception in the Neurotic.* D.Phil. thesis, University of Oxford.

Zeiss, A. M., Lewinsohn, P. M. and Munoz, R. F. (1979). Nonspecific improvement effects in depression using interpersonal skills training, pleasant activity schedules, or cognitive training. *J. Consult. Clin. Psychol.* 47, 427–39.

Zigler, E. and Phillips, L. (1962). Social competence and the process-reactive distinction in psychopathology. *J. Abnorm. Soc. Psychol.* 65, 215–22.

Zimbardo, P. G. (1977). *Shyness.* Reading, Mass.: Addison-Wesley.

8 Methods of social skills training*

MICHAEL ARGYLE

Introduction

Each of the chapters in this book has made some reference to the methods of social skills training (SST) which are being used for the skills described. In this chapter I shall consider these methods in more detail, and in particular discuss the evidence for the effectiveness of each method.

The traditional means of training, or lack of it, was training on the job; that is, simply learning by experience. This came to be supplemented in some cases, like teaching, by assigning an experienced performer of the skill to watch the trainee in action and give him helpful advice. Research into certain skills, like supervising work groups, led to the establishment of a body of knowledge about these skills which was passed on in the 1950s by educational methods, especially lectures and discussions. Developments in the social psychology of groups and the rise of the T-group and encounter-group movements led to the introduction of various kinds of group sensitivity training, especially for managers. Meanwhile role playing had been increasing in popularity and was boosted by the availability of videotape-recorders. It became widely used in assertiveness training and in SST for mental patients. The latest developments in SST are extensions of role playing based on new findings in social psychology – for example, in non-verbal (NV) communication, sequence analysis, and the study of social situations.

Not all of these methods have been found to be successful, and it is

* This chapter also appears in Argyle (ed.) (1981).

important to carry out follow-up studies. In a final section I shall discuss the design of such studies.

Learning on the job

Improvement of social skills by experience occurs mainly as a result of trial-and-error processes, together with the development of larger units of response. Unfortunately this seems to be a very unreliable form of training. A person can do a job for years and never discover the right social skills: some experienced interviewers have great difficulty with candidates who will not talk, for example. Or people can somehow learn the wrong skills by experience: Fiedler (1970) found that the more years of experience industrial supervisors had the *less* effective they were. Argyle, *et al.* (1958) found that supervisors often learnt the *wrong* things by experience, e.g. to use close, punitive and authoritarian styles of supervision.

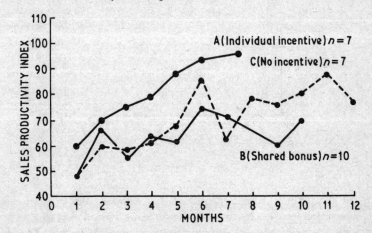

Figure 8.1   Learning curves for selling (from Argyle, *et al.* 1968).

Mary Lydall, Mansur Lalljee and I conducted several studies of the learning of social skills on the job. In one of them an attempt was made to plot the learning curve for selling: this task was chosen because there is an objective criterion of success. Annual fluctuations in trade were overcome by expressing the sales of a beginner as a percentage of the average sales of three experienced sellers in the same department. It was found that there was an overall improvement, especially where there was an individual incentive scheme (Fig. 8.1).

However, individuals responded in a variety of ways and while on average most improved, some did not and others got steadily worse. Again it seems that simply doing the job doesn't always lead to improvement.

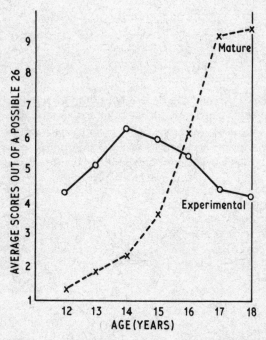

Figure 8.2 Experimental and mature solutions to social problems (from McPhail 1967).

McPhail (1967) studied the process of acquiring social competence during adolescence. He gave problem situations to 100 males and 100 females aged 12–18. Alternative solutions were offered and those chosen were found to change with age in an interesting way (Fig. 8.2). The younger subjects gave a lot of rather crude, aggressive, dominating responses. McPhail classified these as 'experimental' attempts to acquire by trial and error social skills for dealing with the new situations that adolescents face. The older ones, on the other hand, chose more skilful, sophisticated social techniques, similar to those used by adults.

Learning on the job has a great advantage over all other forms of training: there is no problem of transfer from training to real life.

Very often an experienced practitioner is assigned to help the trainee by observing him in action and offering helpful advice. Several studies show that for this kind of coaching and feedback to work, certain conditions must be met:

(1) Clear feedback must be given on what the trainee is doing wrong. Gage *et al.* (1960) asked 3900 schoolchildren to fill in rating scales to describe their ideal teacher and how their actual teachers behaved; the results were shown to half of the teachers, who subsequently improved on ten of the twelve scales, compared with the no-feedback group. This kind of feedback is usually not available.

(2) To improve performance new social techniques must be found. The best way of generating new responses is for an expert to suggest them and to demonstrate them. Learning on the job can be speeded up by imitating successful performers, but it may not be clear exactly what they are doing.

(3) Learning on the job will occur if there is a trainer on the spot who often sees the trainee in action and holds regular feedback and coaching sessions. The trainer should be an expert performer of the skill himself and should be sensitized to the elements and processes of social interaction. The success of such coaching will depend on there being a good relation between the trainee and the supervisor.

Educational (intellectual) methods

For all social skills there is a certain amount of new information and understanding to be acquired. Early attempts to teach, for example, supervisory skills by lecture and discussion were found to have very little effect, so that educational methods were generally abandoned. The motor-skill model suggests that purely intellectual methods would not be much good — you can't learn to swim by reading books about it. However, in cross-cultural training successful use has been made of educational methods alone or in combination with other techniques. This is an area where there is a lot to be learnt about the other culture, its rules, ideas and values.

Reading

This is one of the most widely used methods of education. Many self-improvement books in different areas have been produced, particularly in the USA, such as that by Carnegie (1936) which has been widely read. More recently there have been a number of books on do-it-yourself assertiveness training, e.g. Bower and Bower (1976), though no follow-up studies have been carried out. 'Bibliotherapy' produces short-term benefits at least in a number of areas, including weight reduction, study behaviour, fear reduction and exercise, though often some minimal therapist contact is needed (Glasgow and Rosen 1978). One area of social skills where reading is regularly used is for inter-cultural communication — where, for example, programmed texts based on critical incident surveys in the form of Culture Assimilators have been quite successful (Fiedler, *et al.* 1971). However, in this field it is normal to combine learning by reading with more active forms of training, and self-help manuals usually include guidance on exercises to be carried out. It may be necessary, however, to have someone who can take the role of trainer and give some feedback on performance.

Reading is potentially a very important form of SST, since it is possible to reach many people.

Lectures

Lectures can be given in which various aspects of skill are explained, followed by discussion. They may focus on the basic principles of social behaviour or on the details of recommended social techniques. The lectures may be followed by discussion among the trainees, or there may be guided discussions without lectures. Experience with management training shows that lectures on 'human relations' are often very popular, and are a good means of conveying knowledge, though not a good way of changing attitudes. Can social skills be taught by means of lectures? Follow-up studies show that lectures on human relations lead to improved scores on questionnaires, but it has not been shown that any behavioural changes in skill are produced. There are certain difficulties about lectures. They are no good unless the audience is really interested in what the lecturer has to say, or unless he can make them interested by the forcefulness of his presentation, and unless he has a manner and status which make him personally acceptable.

There is some evidence that *group discussions* on human relations problems, without lectures, lead to changes in questionnaire measures. Group discussion can also be looked at as a kind of role playing of group problem solving; it has been found that it results in improved committee skills (Maier 1953). One problem about group methods is that there may be little input of new information to the group. There can be various degrees of feedback, instruction or other guidance from the trainer; probably the more there is the more successful the results. In so far as the method works, success is partly due to the better assimilation of material put over in lectures or otherwise and through practice in group behaviour. It is also possible for a skilful leader to bring about changes in attitudes and values as a result of discussion.

The case-study method

This has been used for teaching social skills to schoolchildren. A case is presented by the teacher, or from a textbook, which illustrates problems such as dealing with authority, emotional problems at home or moral dilemmas. The case is then discussed by the class under the guidance of the teacher (McPhail 1972).

I shall refer to the use of films for modelling in connection with role playing. A number of suitable films are now available, mainly for management skills. Social skills trainers often make up their own videotapes for modelling behaviour for trainees. However, no follow-up studies are yet available on the use of films for this purpose. Films have been used for training in manual skills for some time, and these are found to be successful under certain conditions: if the learner has to try out part of the skill after each piece of film, if there is discussion before or after the film, if the film is shot from his point of view — e.g. over his shoulder — and if appropriate use is made of slow motion, animation and sequences of stills, showing the successive steps in the skill. Again, it looks as if films can play an important part in an overall training scheme but are not much use alone; and so far there are very few suitable films available.

However, there is some evidence that the combination of these methods, especially of lectures and group methods, can lead to increases in social skill. Sorenson (1958) studied 205 managers before and after such a course, and 267 controls. Ratings by other managers showed that the course trainees were rated as more co-operative, self-confident, poised and higher on 'consideration' (i.e. looking after the welfare of subordinates) and delegation. It is quite likely that neither lectures, reading, nor group discussion alone will do the job, but that together they can be very successful, especially in conveying knowledge about effective skills, understanding of social interaction and general awareness of interpersonal phenomena. On the other hand, managers may be better able than other people to apply on the job new principles that they have learnt.

Training in groups

Therapy groups, T-groups and encounter groups were designed for different forms of training. The only kind of group training which has been recommended by a contributor to these two books is the T-group (Argyle (ed.) 1981, Chapter 5).

T-groups

The members of a T-group spend their time studying the group and the processes of social interaction that take place in it. The trainer typically starts the group off by saying 'My name is _____, and I am the appointed staff trainer of this group and am here to help you in the study of this group as best I can'. T-groups consist of about twelve trainees who meet for a series of two-hour periods, weekly or during a residential course. The T-group sessions are often combined with lectures, role playing and other activities but the T-group is regarded as central.

The topic is unusual: one of the basic rules of T-groups is that conversation must be confined to the 'here and now', i.e. what is happening in the group. The role of the trainer is unusual: he does not take charge or act as a leader, but occasionally intervenes to make interpretations, provide feedback or draw attention to particular problems. He behaves rather like a group therapist, except that he does not discuss the personalities or problems of individuals, but rather the common problems of the group. This abdication of the role of the leader causes some perplexity and annoyance at first: the members are unfamiliar with the situation and seek help from the trainer in coping with it. During the early sessions there is a struggle for dominance, and questions of intimacy and friendship are sorted out. For females in particular it is found that there are problems of dependency – who to be dependent on, and how dependent to be.

Behaviour in T-groups has a strange quality, the conversation is somewhat stilted and embarrassed, and some members either do not take part at all, or couples engage in irrelevant conversation ('pairing'). A curious pattern of role differentiation has been reported in Harvard T-groups, including 'distressed females', who take little part in the conversation, 'paranoid' and 'moralistic' resisters, who oppose the official task, and 'sexual scapegoats' who present their masculinity problems for the group to study (Mann, *et al.* 1967).

One of the main things that the trainer does is to teach people to give and receive feedback, so that members may become aware of the effect of their behaviour on others and find out how others see them. The trainer shows how to make non-evaluative comments on the behaviour of others, and tries to reduce the defensiveness of those whose behaviour is being commented upon. Feedback is provided in other ways; members may take turns to act as observers who later report back to the group, tape-recordings of previous sessions are studied and analyses by professional observers may be presented.

Encounter groups

These use a number of exercises designed to give experience of intimacy and other social relationships. Here is an example of the exercises used at Esalen (Schutz 1967).

To help people who have difficulty in giving or receiving affection or who avoid emotional closeness:

(1) 'Give and take affection'. One person stands in the centre of a circle with his eyes shut; the others approach him and express their feelings towards him non-verbally however they wish — usually by hugging, stroking, massaging, lifting, etc.
(2) 'Roll and rock'. One person stands in the centre of a circle, relaxed and with his eyes shut; the group passes him round from person to person, taking his weight. The group then picks him up and sways him gently backwards and forwards, very quietly.

How successful are T-groups and encounter groups? This is a matter on which there is considerable disagreement. Those who have been in these groups report that they have been through a powerful experience. Smith (1975) reviewed thirty-one controlled follow-up studies, of which twenty-one showed positive results. The effect was greatest on self-reports, rather less on ratings by others or on organizational effectiveness. Most studies have found that the majority are unchanged. The disagreement arises over how many become *worse*. This issue has not yet been resolved. Several studies show a 'casualty rate' of 8 per cent, including the rather careful study by Lieberman, *et al.* (1973), and a number of those reviewed by Hartley, *et al.* (1976). Other studies suggest a lower rate of 1—2 per cent, and this is the figure favoured by Georgiades and Orlans in Argyle (ed.) (1981) Chapter 5. It is agreed, however, that the rate of disturbance is highest with certain kinds of trainer, especially those who encourage confrontation and the expression of anger.

Some people may go to groups as a last resort before seeing a psychiatrist, some may become worse as a result of other changes in their lives. It has been said in defence of T-groups that they may be the only way of dealing with particularly difficult members of staff — who are reformed or never seen again. A problem with encounter groups which use a lot of bodily contact is that some clients end up with a different spouse from the one they started with. Some people enjoy the groups so much that they lose interest in ordinary life and want to spend all of their time having 'deep and meaningful experiences' in groups.

In a later section I shall discuss the need to accompany SST with various aspects of personal growth, such as increased self-confidence, reduced anxiety and new ideas and principles. Part of the attraction of group methods is that they provide opportunity for group discussion, self-disclosure of anxiety and thrashing out general problems connected with the job. However, I do not believe that the special procedures used in T-groups or encounter groups are what is needed. It might be better to have a series of group discussions led by a sympathetic and experienced leader who is familiar with the problems of young doctors, social workers, etc., and who can help them make the necessary emotional and cognitive changes.

Role playing

Most forms of SST are varieties of role playing. Role playing consists of trying out a social skill away from the real situation in the laboratory, clinic or training centre on other trainees or role partners provided for the purpose. The training usually consists of a series of sessions which may last from 1 to 3 hours, depending on the size and stamina of the group. In each session a particular aspect of the skill or a particular range of problem situations is dealt with. There are three main phases to role-playing exercises:

(1) There is a lecture, discussion, demonstration, tape-recording or a film about a particular aspect of the skill. This is particularly important when an unfamiliar skill is being taught or when rather subtle social techniques are used. The demonstration is important: this is known as 'modelling'.

(2) A problem situation is defined and stooges are produced for trainees to role play with for 7–15 minutes each. The background to the situation may be filled in with written materials, such as the application forms of candidates for interview, or background information about personnel problems – the stooges may be carefully trained beforehand to provide various problems, such as talking too much or having elaborate but plausible excuses. It is found in microteaching that it is better to use real pupils than other trainee teachers as stooges, although this is a lot more trouble to arrange; the same probably applies to other areas of SST.

(3) There is a feedback session, consisting of verbal comments by the trainer, discussion with the other trainees, and playback of audio- or videotapes. Verbal feedback is used to draw attention, constructively and tactfully, to what the trainee was doing wrong and to suggest alternative styles of behaviour. The tape-recordings provide clear evidence for the accuracy of what is being said.

(4) There is often a fourth phase, in which the role-playing is repeated. In microteaching this is known as 're-teaching'.

There are a number of practical difficulties in conducting role playing, which are discussed in the chapter on social work skills (p. 128). Trainees have to be given the right attitude to the training: it should be enjoyable and carried out sufficiently light-heartedly for them not to be embarrassed, but it should also be seen as a serious exercise, and they should not 'ham it up'. They may also need to be introduced gradually to the idea of videotaping.

Follow-up studies have found that role playing combined with coaching, feedback and modelling is successful with many kinds of professional clients and mental patients, and that it is one of the most successful forms of SST for all of these groups.

Feedback

This is one of the crucial components. It can be provided in several ways. It may come from the other members of the group, either in free discussion, discussion in smaller groups, questionnaires, or behavioural checklists. This must be done carefully or it will be disturbing to the recipients of the feedback; on the other hand, it is probably a valuable part of the training process for those observing.

It may be given by the trainer, who should be in a position to give expert guidance on the social techniques which are effective, and who may be able to increase sensitivity to the subtler nuances of inter-action. He may correct errors − such as interrupting, looking or sounding unfriendly. He can suggest alternative social techniques, such as ways of dealing with awkward clients or situations. This has to be done very carefully: the trainer's remarks should be gentle and kind enough not to upset, but firm and clear enough to have some effect.

Audiotape-recordings may be taken and played back to the trainee immediately after his performance. I have found that it is better for the trainer's comments to precede the playback so that trainees know what to look for.

Videotape-recordings can be used in a similar way: the videotape is played back to the trainee after his performance. This directs the trainee's attention to the behavioural (facial, bodily and gestural) aspects of his performance as well as to the auditory. It may be useful to play back the sound-tape separately to focus attention on sound.

It is usual for trainers to be generally encouraging and also reward-ing for specific aspects of behaviour, though there is little experi-mental evidence for the value of such reinforcement. It is common to combine role playing with modelling and video playback, both of which are discussed below.

Modelling

Modelling can consist of demonstrations by one of the therapists, or the showing of films or videotapes. It is used when it is difficult to teach the patient by verbal description alone. This applies to complex skills for neurotic or volunteer clients, and to simpler skills for more disturbed patients and children. It is generally used in conjunction with role playing between role-play sessions and is accompanied by verbal instructions, i.e. coaching.

The success of modelling has been found to vary between different groups. For children it is the best technique (e.g. O'Connor 1972). For inpatients it is an essential part of SST − though the effectiveness of SST for these patients is in some doubt (p. 176). On the other hand, a number of outpatient studies have obtained good results without modelling (e.g. Argyle, *et al.* 1974), while McFall and Twentyman (1973) found that modelling made no contribution to assertiveness training for students, perhaps because they knew what to do already.

Modelling has been found to be most effective when the model is similar to the trainees, e.g. in age; when the model shows 'coping' rather than 'mastery' (i.e. is not too expert); when there is a verbal narrative, labelling the model's behaviour; when the model is warm and preferably live, with multiple models; and when the model's behaviour is seen to lead to favourable consequences (Thelen, *et al.* 1979).

Video playback

This is widely used in conjunction with role playing. Bailey and Sowder (1970) and Griffiths (1974) have reviewed some of the studies comparing the effectiveness of role playing with and without video, and came to the conclusion that there is little evidence for its usefulness. In fact nearly all the studies cited showed that patients did better when video playback was used. A later, carefully designed study on people who replied to an advertisement for SST obtained clearly better results with video; the criterion measure consisted of blind ratings of role playing (Maxwell 1976). Video playback may not be equally suitable for all kinds of patients. Sarason and Ganzer (1973) believe that it should not be used with extremely anxious or self-conscious patients. Most people find it mildly disturbing at first, and that it increases self-consciousness; however this wears off by the second or third session. The author has found it particularly useful in training NV behaviour.

'Homework'

How do patients apply what they have learned in the training setting to real life? The main solution so far has been via 'homework'. Trainees are asked to try out the skills which they have just learnt several times before the next weekly session and to report back on any difficulties. They may be given written notes on the exercises to be carried out, and the steps in each, and they may be asked to keep notes of what happened. Falloon, *et al.* (1977) found that outpatients who were given structured homework assignments did better on nearly all outcome measures. There is usually difficulty in persuading patients to do the homework, however. This can be done by the use of token rewards, or by refusing to continue treatment until homework assignments have been completed.

Lindsay (1980) increased the generalization of conversational skills in schizophrenics, from clinic to ward, by using token rewards for homework. Matson, *et al.* (1980) selected for training those target behaviours which the nursing staff were willing to reinforce on the ward, such as talking clearly, being cheerful, complying with requests and appropriate NV communication.

These and other studies show that homework is a useful way of producing memorization.

Individual or group methods?

Most therapists and other trainers take clients in groups of 6–12, since groups have the advantage of providing a ready-made social situation and a series of role partners, make more economical use of therapist time and enable patients to feel more at ease in the company of other similar people. On the other hand, groups of patients contain bad models, so there should be more than one trainer present, and it is difficult to concentrate on individual problems. One solution is to start patients in groups but also to give them some individual sessions for particular problems. Very disturbed or regressed patients should be taken individually (Trower, *et al.* 1978). There is no problem in using groups for professional SST.

Interviewer training

One of the first social skills to be taught by role playing was selection interviewing. In the course for selection interviewing devised by Sidney and Argyle (1969) some of the exercises were designed to teach participants how to deal with 'awkward' candidates. Trainees interview trained stooges who talk too much, too little, are nervous, bombastic, anxious and so on. Each role-playing session on this course begins with a lecture and a film about the problems to be role played. There is also training in how to assess stability, judgment, achievement,

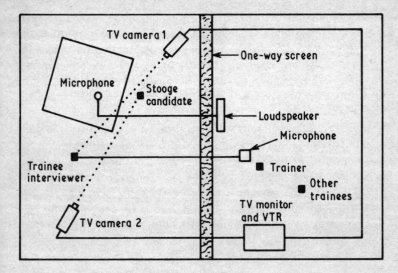

Figure 8.3 Laboratory arrangements for interviewer training (from Argyle 1968). VTR = videotape recorder.

motivation, etc. in the interview and how to avoid common errors of person perception.

Role playing can be conducted without the use of any specialized equipment but it is greatly assisted if certain laboratory arrangements are available. An ideal set-up for interviewer training is shown in Figure 8.3. The role playing takes place on one side of a one-way screen and is observed by the trainer and other trainees. A videotape is taken of the role playing. The trainer is able to communicate with the role player through an ear-microphone; the trainer can give comments and suggestions to the trainee while the role playing is proceeding. (I once had to advise an interviewer trainee dealing with an over-amorous 'candidate' to move his seat back 3 feet.)

Microteaching

This is now widely used for training teachers. A trainee teacher prepares a short lesson, and teaches five or six children for 10–15 minutes; this is followed by videotape playback and comments by the trainer, after which the trainee teaches the same lesson again. There are usually a number of sessions, each being devoted to one particular teaching skill: asking higher-order questions, encouraging pupil participation, explaining clearly with examples, etc. This form of training is found to be very much faster than alternative forms of training and is probably the best way of eliminating bad teaching habits (Brown 1975, Peck and Tucker 1973).

Management skills

Rackham and Morgan (1977) have developed a set of procedures for training in committee work, chairmanship, selling and related skills. They use a set of categories, which is modified for particular skills, containing items such as content proposals, procedural proposals, building, supporting, disagreeing, defending/attacking, testing understanding, summarizing, seeking information, giving information (the Chairman list). Good and bad performers at the skill are nominated and their rates of using the categories compared. Trainees learn the use of the categories and participate in role-play exercises while observers record how often they use the categories. The trainer then gives feedback, consisting of information about each trainee's score on the categories, which are compared with the rates for the good performers. Follow-up studies have shown positive results, though these studies were not very carefully controlled.

Special training methods

Some forms of SST have drawn heavily on the results of research in social psychology, and this is particularly the case with the Oxford form of SST. It has been found that facial expression, tone of voice, and other aspects of NVC communication make a major contribution to social competence (p. 10), and that trainees often need to improve their performance in this sphere. Here are some examples, related to the processes described earlier.

Expression of NV signals

In training mental patients it is common to coach them in NV communication, since they are often very inexpressive in this sphere, or send NV messages which are hostile rather than friendly. Study of a patient's role-played performance in the clinic shows which NV signals require training, though the commonest ones are face and voice. Facial expression can be trained with the help of a mirror and later with a videotape-recorder. Trainees are asked to take part in short conversations, while expressing certain emotions in the face: sad, happy, etc. If there is difficulty in producing the correct expression in all parts of the face the photographs by Ekman and Friesen (1975) can be used as models. The voice can be trained with the help of an audiotape-recorder; trainees are asked to read passages from the paper in friendly, dominant, surprised, etc. tones of voice, and these are then played back and discussed. Details of correct vocal qualities for these emotions are given in Scherer (1979). I have found that neurotic patients improve rapidly with training. In other kinds of training there are always a few clients who need some help in this sphere. In most skills it is important to indicate attitudes such as warmth or concern, which require the right NV signals.

Perceptual training

It may also be necessary to train people in the perception of NV signals. Some convicts, for example, can't tell when people are becoming upset, so that fights start (p. 169). For professional skills like social work and psychotherapy it is important to be able to judge the emotional states of others. The Ekman and Friesen (1975) photographs can be used to train people to decode facial expression. Trainees can be taught to decode tones of voice by listening to tape-recordings of neutral messages produced in different emotional states (Davitz 1964). In each case it is easy to test the subject, for example by finding out the percentage of recordings which they can decode correctly.

Jecker, *et al.* (1965) succeeded in training teachers to perceive more accurately whether or not pupils had understood what they were being taught. The measure consisted of a series of one-minute films showing children being taught; a subsequent question to the child (not shown in the film) found out if he really had understood or not. By showing teachers these films, and by drawing attention to the behavioural cues for comprehension, it was possible to increase their scores on a new set of similar films. A number of studies of teacher training have found that training in observation skills and practice with the Flanders category scheme improves teaching skills (Peck and Tucker 1973). This is probably because teachers become sensitized to the importance of pupil participation and the need to ask questions; they would already be able to perform the skilled moves which were needed.

Planning and the use of feedback

The social skills model (p. 2) suggests some further points at which training can be useful. A common problem with mental patients is a failure to pursue persistent goals and a tendency to react passively to others. Assertiveness training is also directed at making the trainees take more initiative and pursue their goals. We have used special exercises for this problem; trainees are asked to carry out a simple skill, like interviewing, which requires that they take the initiative throughout. They can plan the encounter and take notes; the trainer communicates with an ear-microphone during the role playing if the performer runs out of conversation.

The social skill model also emphasizes the importance of responding to feedback. The social survey interview was given as an example earlier (p. 18): if the respondent does not produce the desired information, revised questions are asked until this information is produced. The selection interview provides another example: the interviewer has to use different styles of behaviour with different interviewees. If a candidate does not talk enough the interviewer asks more open-ended questions, waits for the answers, and gives positive reinforcement for whatever is said. If the candidate talks too much, is very nervous, boastful, etc., other techniques are required.

Conversational sequences

All social skills use conversation, i.e. a sequence of utterances, and the control of sequences is an important part of the skill. Some neurotic patients are virtually incapable of sustaining a conversation at all (p. 173). Teachers need to be able to control such cycles of interaction as teacher lectures → teacher asks question → pupil replies (p. 17), and other longer cycles. During such repeated sequences there is also a build-up in the complexity of the topic being taught. The selection interview is similar: there is a certain structure of questions—answers—modified and follow-up questions, and a structure of episodes and sub-episodes, based on topics and sub-topics. Every social skill uses certain conversational sequences, which can be learned. And every social skill has a number of difficulties in this sphere, for which the solution can be taught. Salesmen may have difficulty in controlling interaction with the client; doctors may find it is hard to terminate encounters; survey interviewers may have to deal with respondents who wander off the point.

Situational analysis

Some mental patients and many ordinary adults have difficulty in coping with specific social situations. In a number of professional social skills the performer has to deal with a variety of situations, as in the cases of social workers and supervisors. It would be possible to include in the training some analysis of the main situations involved, and especially of those which are found difficult, in terms of goals and goal structure, rules, roles, etc. (p. 21). Situational analysis has been used in the treatment of obesity, by discovering the situations in which over-eating occurs, and the series of events leading up to it (Ferguson 1975). A similar approach is commonly used in the treatment of alcoholics.

Taking the role of the other

Chandler (1973) succeeded in improving ability to see the other's point of view (and reducing delinquency) by means of exercises in which groups of five young delinquents developed and made video-recordings of skits about relevant real-life situations, in which each member of the group played a part.

Self-presentation

In addition to the usual role-playing exercises, trainees can be given advice over clothes, hair and other aspects of appearance. Their voices can be trained to produce a more appropriate accent or tone of voice. There is a correlation between physical attractiveness and mental health (p. 28), and some therapeutic success has been obtained by improving the appearance of patients. The recidivism of male criminals has been reduced by removing tattooing and scars (p. 179).

Some problems of social skills training

Prerequisites for successful training

To carry out role-playing or most other forms of training it is necessary to have a working vocabulary of the main elements in the repertoire for the skill being taught. This is needed to communicate with trainees, to label their behaviour, and for them to monitor their own performance. A vocabulary is needed in the following areas:

(1) Speech acts, e.g. makes interpretation, reflects feelings.
(2) Speech contents, e.g. candidate's exam results, leisure activities, future plans.
(3) NV communication, e.g. smiles, nods head.
(4) Actions, e.g. takes temperature, looks at tongue.

The same NV signals are used in all skills, though some will be more common in a particular case. Bales (1950) produced what was intended to be a universal set of twelve speech acts, but later work in particular fields has led to the development of categories tailored to the special needs of teaching, psychotherapy, etc. In some fields, however, there are a number of different category schemes, reflecting the ideas and interests of different investigators or trainers. A very large number of systems are used for training teachers, for example (Simon and Boyer 1974).

A second prerequisite is knowledge of the skills which are most successful. Without such knowledge the trainer has to fall back on common sense, which is very fallible in this field. Each of the chapters in this book has indicated the extent of research on the optimum skills, and it is clearly less extensive in some areas than others. A serious problem is that the most effective social skill may vary with situational factors such as characteristics of the others being handled; this has been studied most in the case of supervisory skills. The best skills may also be different in different classes, races or other sub-cultures. This is a particular problem with training mental patients, since the skills which they should be taught may vary considerably with their social class, etc.; and very often this kind of knowledge is not yet available.

Transfer to real life

Training on the job is the only form of training which does not have to face the problem of transferring the skills which have been learnt in training centre, lab or clinic to the real world. T-groups are very different from the outside world and it has been said that all they train for is other T-groups. Role playing usually tries to deal with this problem by means of 'homework' (p. 199); however, trainees are often reluctant to try the new skills out or may refuse to do so. Some role playing uses quite realistic simulations of the real situations; examples are the model villages constructed in the Caribbean and Hawaii for preparing members of the Peace Corps for Latin America and the Far East (Guthrie 1966). There are other ways of preparing trainees for varied and unexpected incidents in real life. More abstract principles of behaviour may be taught, as opposed to specific skills. An example is 'be rewarding', where this can take a variety of forms. Another is to learn to watch out for feedback and to take rapid corrective action. If trainees learn the basic principles of situational analysis they can be on the look out for the particular rules, roles and other features of totally new situations. It is also possible to acquire the habit of learning new social skills whenever these are needed — by imitation of successful performers, and studying the behaviour which is effective and ineffective.

There may be resistance to trying out new social skills because it is feared they will be found surprising by friends and colleagues and will be rejected. Sending managers off to a remote training course is often unsuccessful for this reason. The solution is to carry out training within the organization and to show that senior members are in support of the behaviour being advocated by using them as trainers in some way. Some forms of SST for patients use their friends or family in the training in the same way (p. 180).

The search for more economical methods

If most professional people, many mental patients and perhaps 10 per cent of the normal population need, or could profit by, SST, who is going to administer it? The use of group methods is common, because it saves trainer time and provides role partners. What of do-it-yourself methods? We have seen that 'bibliotherapy' can be useful, if combined with more acted methods.

Some microteaching has been carried out without trainers: trainees simply record and play back videotapes of their own role playing and compare them with films of model teachers. However, microteaching is more successful when there is a trainer (Peck and Tucker 1973).

Another method is simply to arrange for clients to have practice encounters with one another without a trainer. Arkowitz has found that this is successful in improving subjective feelings of confidence and reducing anxiety after six practice dates (Arkowitz, *et al.* 1978), or twelve practice interactions with potential same-sex friends (Royce and Arkowitz 1978). However, although subjective feelings were improved, there was no observed improvement in social skill.

The need for other aspects of personal growth

For several skills it is not enough simply to learn the correct social moves, or it may be impossible to use these skills unless certain emotional problems have been dealt with. Some skill situations commonly arouse anxiety — for example public speaking, dealing with hostile people or opposing others. Learning effective skills is certainly part of the answer and practising the skill successfully helps but may not be sufficient. Performers may simply lack the self-confidence to take the responsibilities required, for example, by doctors and social workers. This entails a change in self-image, which is usually produced by simply doing the job. Training courses often include an element of guided group discussion, which can help trainees to talk about these matters, and receive some social support. Newcomers to a social role often need some new set of ideas or principles which will help them to deal with the moral, political or wider (even philosophical issues) at stake: for example, doctors may be concerned about how long to keep patients alive, social workers about conflicts between the demands of law and the interests of clients. Again, this goes beyond social skills and can be tackled by guided group discussion, together with reflecting on the experience of performing the skill.

Methods of assessing training procedures

The assessment of social competence

Any assessment of the effectiveness of SST requires some means of measuring the social competence of individuals.

Objective assessment of competence   The best way of measuring social competence is by a performer's success in attaining the goals of the job or situation which he is in. The competence of a salesperson, for example, could be measured by his average level of sales over a period of time compared with others' selling in the same department. In practice there are often complications; in the sales cases there may be informal rules to the effect that the senior salesperson deals with customers first, or deals with more expensive items. There may be more than one index of success: for example, the supervisor of a working group is trying to maximize the quantity and quality of output, and to keep down absenteeism, labour turnover and accidents. If such indices have low or negative correlations with each other it is necessary to weight them or decide on cut-off points for acceptable performance. Again it may be difficult to compare different supervisors since there are other differences between their departments; for example, in the nature of the work and the characteristics of their working groups. Some of these difficulties are less important in follow-up studies, since these study *differences* before and after training in the same departments.

Assessing the competence of patients, or of otherwise normal adults or children in everyday non-work settings is more difficult. It is easier to recognize failures or skill rather than success: the extent to which an individual cannot communicate clearly or effectively, cannot establish or maintain relationships, quarrels and annoys other people or finds social situations difficult and stressful. However, success can also be assessed by self-ratings, or ratings by others.

Ratings Many follow-up studies have used ratings by the supervisors of those being trained or by colleagues. There may be ratings on a number of different aspects of performance, including competence in several sub-tasks or situations. Such ratings are more useful if the supervisor sees the trainee in action on several occasions, though this is not entirely satisfactory since the trainee may perform differently when watched. Raters may be subject to various kinds of error in the use of rating scales, such as halo effect and central tendency. Ratings are not very satisfactory for before-and-after studies, since the attitudes of raters towards the method of training may affect their willingness to indicate improvement or deterioration after training.

Subjective reports These have been widely used in psychiatric SST, and are acceptable there since one of the goals of training is to modify subjective feelings of anxiety and discomfort. Self-reports of competence are much less satisfactory; trainees can learn the right answers without their behaviour being affected at all (Fleishman, *et al.* 1955). And asking people how much they enjoyed a training course is of very little value — they usually say they enjoyed it very much. The use of rating scales and tests with patients was described earlier (p. 161).

Role-played tests   I have said that role-played tests for assertiveness in mental patients have been found to have rather low validity (p. 162). For all role-played tests it is probably necessary to sample a number of tasks, and to ensure that these are similar to real life. Such tests have been used in a number of studies, and have the advantage over objective measues of providing exactly the same situation for all trainees. In a follow-up study the pre-test provides some practice, so that an untrained control group is essential. The use of staged events for role-play tests was described earlier (p. 162).

Other measures   I have discussed some specialized forms of training which focus on particular aspects of performance, and hence may require measures of special aspects of social competence. Examples are accuracy of perception, level of anxiety, and voice quality. On the other hand, improving such specific aspects of social performance is no use unless it increases overall social competence.

The design of follow-up studies

The most obvious procedure is to compare the competence of trainees before and after training. The difficulty with this design is that with the passage of time other changes may affect them and they may improve anyway through being more familiar with the test situation (for some kinds of measure). Many investigators have used the before-and-after study with control groups of similar but untrained individuals. In practice it may be difficult to find a suitable control group. Why were the trainees being trained but not the members of the control group? Perhaps the trainees were in greater need of training. A design which avoids this is the after-only design, which compares people after a period of training, after different kinds of training or after no training. Members of the control group may be scheduled for training at a later date. This method, however, requires very careful matching of the groups of individuals to be compared and needs larger numbers.

Sometimes, it would be unacceptable to withhold training for a control group, for example with patients. One procedure here is the cross-over design in which two groups of trainees receive treatments A and B, or treatment and no treatment, in reverse order (Argyle, *et al.* 1974). Another method is the multiple baseline procedure for follow-up of individuals in intensive clinical trials, which was described earlier (p. 176).

References

Argyle, M., (ed.) (1981). *Social Skills and Work*. London: Methuen.

Argyle, M., Bryant, B. and Trower, P. (1974). Social skills training and psychotherapy: a comparative study. *Psychol. Med.* 4, 435–43.

Argyle, M., Gardner, G. and Cioffi, F. (1958). Supervisory methods related to productivity, absenteeism and labour turnover. *Hum. Relat.* 11, 23–45.

Argyle, M., Lalljee, M. G. and Lydall, M. (1968). Selling as a social skill (mimeo).

Arkowitz, H. (1977). Measurement and modification of minimal dating behavior. *In* Hersen, M. (ed.). *Progress in Behavior Modification 5*. New York: Academic Press.

Arkowitz, H., Hinton, R., Perl, J. and Himadi, W. (1978). Treatment strategies for dating anxiety in college men based on real-life practice. *Counseling Psychol.* 7, 41–6.

Bailey, K. G. and Sowder, W. T. (1970). Audiotape and videotape self-confrontation in psychotherapy. *Psychol. Bull.* 74, 27–137.

Bales, R. F. (1950). *Interaction Process Analysis*. Cambridge, Mass.: Addison-Wesley.

Bower, S. A. and Bower, G. H. (1976). *Asserting yourself*. Reading, Mass.: Addison-Wesley.

Brown, G. (1975). *Microteaching*. London: Methuen.

Carnegie, D. (1936). *How to Win Friends and Influence People*. New York: Simon and Schuster.

Chandler, M. J. (1973). Egocentrism and anti-social behavior: the assessment and training of social perspective-taking skills. *Dev. Psychol.* 9, 326–32.

Davitz, J. R. (1964). *The Communication of Emotional Meaning*. New York: McGraw-Hill.

Ekman, P. and Friesen, W. V. (1975). *Unmasking the Face*. Englewood Cliffs: Prentice-Hall.

Falloon, I. R. H., Lindley, P., McDonald, R. and Marks, I. M. (1977). Social skills training of out-patient groups: a controlled study of rehearsal and homework. *Br. J. Psychiatr.* 131, 599–609.

Ferguson, J. M. (1975). *Learning to Eat: Behavior Modification for Weight Control*. New York: Hawthorn Books.

Fiedler, F. E. (1970). Leadership experience and leader effectiveness – another hypothesis shot to hell. *Org. Behav. Hum. Perf.* 5, 1–14.

Fiedler, F. E., Mitchell, R. and Triandis, H. C. (1971). The culture assimilator: an approach to cross-cultural training, *J. Appl. Psychol.* 55, 95–102.

Fleishman, E. A., Harris, E. F. and Burtt, H. E. (1955). *Leadership and Supervision in Industry*. New York: Columbia University Press.

Gage, N. L., Runkel, P. J. and Chatterjee, B. B. (1960). *Equilibrium Theory* and Behavior Change: an Experiment in Feedback from Pupils to Teachers. Urbana, Ill.: Bureau of Educational Research.

Glasgow, R. E. and Rosen, G. M. (1978). Behavioral bibliotherapy: a review of self-help behavior therapy manuals. *Psychol. Bull.* 85, 1–23.

Griffiths, R. D. P. (1974). Videotape feedback as a therapeutic technique: retrospect and prospect. *Behav. Res. Ther.* 12, 1–8.

Gudykunst, W. B., Hammer, M. R. and Wiseman, R. L. (1979). An analysis of an integrated approach to cross-cultural training. *Int. J. Intercultural Rel.* 1, 99–110.

Guthrie, G. M. (1966). Cultural preparation for the Philippines. *In* Textor, R. B. (ed.). *Cultural Frontiers of the Peace Corps.* Cambridge, Mass.: M.I.T. Press.

Hartley, D., Roback, H. B. and Abramowitz, S. I. (1976). Deterioration effects in encounter groups. *Am. Psychol.* 31, 247–55.

Jecker, J. D., Maccoby, N. and Breitrose, H. S. (1965). Improving accuracy in interpreting non-verbal cues of comprehension. *Psychol. Schools* 2, 239–44.

Lieberman, M. A., Yalom, I. D. and Miles, M. B. (1973). *Encounter Groups: First Facts.* New York: Basic Books.

Lindsay, W. R. (1980). The training and generalization of conversation behaviours in psychiatric in-patients: a controlled study employing multiple measures across settings. *Br. J. Soc. Clin. Psychol.* 19, 85–98.

McFall, R. M. and Twentyman, C. T. (1973). Four experiments on the relative contribution of rehearsal, modeling, and coaching to assertive training. *J. Abnorm. Psychol.* 81, 199–218.

McPhail, P. (1967). The development of social skill in adolescents, paper to British Psychological Society (unpublished), Department of Education/ University of Oxford.

McPhail, P. (1972). *Moral Education in Secondary Schools.* London: Longmans.

Maier, N. R. F. (1953). An experimental test of the effect of training on discussion leadership. *Hum. Rel.* 6, 161–73.

Mann, R. D., Gibbard, G. S. and Hartman, J. J. (1967). *Interpersonal Styles and Group Development.* New York: Wiley.

Matson, J. L., Zeiss, A., Zeiss, R. A. and Bowman, W. (1980). A comparison of social skills training and contingent attention to improve behavioural deficits in psychiatric patients. *Br. J. Soc. Clin. Psychol.* 19, 57–72.

Maxwell, S. (1976). An evaluation of social skills training. (Unpublished), University of Otago, Dunedin.

O'Connor, R. D. (1972). Relative efficacy of modeling, shaping, and the combined procedures for modification of social withdrawal. *J. Abnorm. Psychol.* 79, 327–34.

Peck, R. F. and Tucker, J. A. (1973). Research on teacher education. *In* Travers, R. M. W. (ed.). *Second Handbook of Research on Teaching.* Chicago: Rand McNally.

Rackham, N. and Morgan, T. (1977). *Behaviour Analysis and Training.* London: McGraw-Hill.

Royce, W. S. and Arkowitz, H. (1978). Multimodal evaluation of practice interactions as treatment for social isolation. *J. Consult. Clin. Psychol.* 46, 239–45.

Sarason, I. G. and Ganzer, V. J. (1971). *Modeling: an Approach to the Rehabilitation of Juvenile Offenders*. Baltimore, M.D.: U.S. Departments of Health, Education and Welfare.

——— and ——— (1973). Modeling and group discussion in the rehabilitation of juvenile delinquents. *J. Counseling Psychol.* 20, 442–9.

Scherer, K. R. (1979). Nonlinguistic indicators of emotion and psychopathology. *In* Izard, C. E. (ed.). *Emotion in Personality and Psychopathology*. New York: Plenum, pp. 495–529.

Schutz, W. C. (1958). *FIRO: A Three-Dimensional Theory of Interpersonal Behavior*. New York: Holt, Rinehart and Winston.

——— (1967). An evaluation of social skills training. (Unpublished). University of Otago, Dunedin.

Sidney, E. and Argyle, M. (1969). *Training in Selection Interviewing*. London: Mantra.

Simon, A. and Boyer, E. G. (eds) (1974). *Mirrors for Behavior, Classroom Interaction Newsletter*. Wyncote, Penn.: Communication Materials Center, 3rd edn.

Smith, P. B. (1975). Controlled studies of the outcome of sensitivity training. *Psychol. Bull.* 82, 597–622.

Sorensen, O. (1958). *The Observed Changes Enquiry*. New York: G.E.C.

Textor, R. B. (ed.) (1966). *Cultural Frontiers of the Peace Corps*. Cambridge, Mass.: M.I.T. Press.

Thelen, M. H., Fry, R. A., Fehrenback, P. A. and Frantschl, N. M. (1979). Therapeutic videotape and film modelling: a review. *Psychol. Bull.* 86, 701–20.

Trower, P., Bryant, B. and Argyle, M. (1978). *Social Skills and Mental Health*. London: Methuen.

Name index

Page numbers in italic type refer to the full reference given at the end of each chapter.

Subject index